ELIMINATION DIETS

AND

THE PATIENT'S ALLERGIES

A HANDBOOK OF ALLERGY

BY

ALBERT H. ROWE, M.D.

LECTURER IN MEDICINE, UNIVERSITY OF CALIFORNIA MEDICAL SCHOOL, SAN FRAN-
CISCO, CALIFORNIA; CONSULTANT IN ALLERGIC DISEASES, ALAMEDA
COUNTY HOSPITAL, OAKLAND, CALIFORNIA

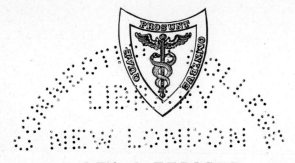

LEA & FEBIGER
PHILADELPHIA

Copyright
LEA & FEBIGER
1941

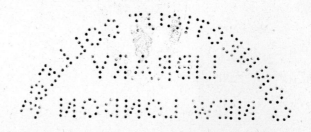

PRINTED IN U. S. A.

TO

HERBERT WILLIAM ALLEN, M.D.

CLINICAL PROFESSOR OF MEDICINE
UNIVERSITY OF CALIFORNIA MEDICAL SCHOOL
TEACHER AND FRIEND

PREFACE

THE use of diet trial in the study of patients with possible food allergy has gained increasing importance as a diagnostic test whenever food allergy is suspected. The frequency of negative skin reactions, especially by the scratch tests, to foods productive of clinical allergy and the occurrence of positive reactions by the scratch and especially by the intradermal tests which are non-specific or only indicate past or potential allergy, justify the use of such diet trial in most patients suspected of food allergy. Moreover, when definite skin reactions are obtained, the reacting foods must be fed to the symptom-free patient at times for days or even longer to determine whether they actually produce clinical allergy. Thus *diet trial at all times is necessary for the determination of clinical food allergies.*

For such diet trial, the writer has found his elimination diets of increasing value during the last fifteen years. In the hands of many physicians, they have become a standardized method for study. Since they exclude most of the foods which commonly produce allergy, their use is more logical than is the sole exclusion of wheat, milk, and eggs. Moreover, the diets list only those foods which are allowed, and carefully arranged menus and directions for their use are contained especially in this publication which will protect nutrition and proper weight maintenance.

Failure to use trial diet as a usual routine when food allergy is suspected often prevents the recognition and relief of its many manifestations. The fear of nutritional damage from diet trial has often prevented adequate use of such dieting. As discussed in this book, test negative diets especially are prone to lead to undernutrition unless menus are carefully arranged to prevent such a result. With the elimination diets, however, and the writer's insistence on maintenance of nutrition, there is no contraindication to the routine and sufficient use of diet trial. *These diets should be used as diagnostic tools as are blood counts and other laboratory tests.*

(5)

Their use implies that the physician suspects and has not *a priori* diagnosed the presence of food allergy.

In the last few years, *the writer has found his cereal-free elimination diet of greatest value because of the frequency of group sensitization to several of the cereal grains.* The diet including rice, corn, and rye (Diets 1 and 2) is of second choice; if allergy to legumes is suspected by history or skin testing it may be initially prescribed at this time. *New detailed menus* with several choices of foods which furnish adequate nutrition have been prepared. Detailed menus for the elimination diets for those patients who must eat away from home are presented. The *fruit-free elimination diets* and their menus, especially important in the study of patients with urticaria, bladder allergy, canker sores, colitis, and other gastro-intestinal symptoms, low calory menus for *obese patients* with actual or suspected food allergy, menus for *diabetic patients* who may be affected with food allergy, and finally suggestions about supplemental elimination diets for the minority of patients who have possible allergy to the foods in the routine elimination diets, have been included in this volume. *Many of the recipes,* especially for the soy, lima, and potato bakery products are new or revised according to the experience of various patients and of my dietitian, Eva Court.

With these more detailed elimination diets and the new recipes and the discussion of the use of such diets in this volume, the routine use of them in the study of patients suspected of food sensitizations is facilitated. The physician himself can give the menus of the diet he advises to the patient; or his office nurse or dietitian, and the dietitians in hospitals or clinics can provide the patient with such menus or prepare the actual meals according to the order of the physician. The method of prescribing the various elimination diets is discussed on page 144.

The necessity of protecting nutrition with adequate protein, calories, vitamins, and minerals has been reiterated throughout this book. This is necessary because of the frequent necessity of adhering to an elimination diet for two or more weeks before evidence of relief of allergy occurs. At times the diet must be followed for months before the changes in the tissues produced by chronic food allergy are relieved so that effective cellular function is restored.

The chapters on Diagnosis, Causes of Allergy and Their Control and the Manifestations of Allergy, include a summary of most of the knowledge at present available concerning these problems. For more detailed information, the various textbooks on allergy (page 257) must be consulted. Inhalant, contactant, and infectant allergies have received attention in this handbook, commensurate with their importance. Inhalant and food allergies hold about equal importance in the production of symptoms in the writer's experience.

The detailed directions in the appendix for the administration of serum especially to patients who have mild or severe allergy thereto are written from the viewpoint of the allergist.

I am indebted to Dr. Carl L. Mauser for the clinical study and treatment of many of our patients, to Jane Hyde for her able supervision of the making of antigens and the skin testing of patients, and to Lucille Chandler for her valuable aid in the preparation and typing of this manuscript. I especially thank Eva Court whose experience in dietetics has rendered valued help in the preparation of the menus and recipes for my elimination diets.

ALBERT H. ROWE.

CONTENTS

CHAPTER I

ELIMINATION, TEST NEGATIVE AND OTHER TRIAL DIETS

CHAPTER II

DIAGNOSIS OF ALLERGY

CHAPTER III

CAUSES OF ALLERGY AND THEIR CONTROL

CHAPTER IV

CLINICAL ALLERGY AND ITS CONTROL

CHAPTER V

THE ELIMINATION DIETS

CHAPTER VI

APPENDIX

ELIMINATION DIETS AND THE PATIENT'S ALLERGIES

CHAPTER I

ELIMINATION, TEST NEGATIVE AND OTHER TRIAL DIETS

The Elimination Diets have been devised for the diagnostic study by physicians, of possible food allergy in patients suffering with symptoms which with varying frequency arise from food allergy. They were first proposed by the writer in 1926 and revised in 1933, and *contain those foods which infrequently produce clinical allergy.* These foods have been determined by skin reactions, by histories of food idiosyncrasies, and by trial diets, the allergenic activity of such foods being finally checked by the actual production of the symptoms by the eating of the foods in question. *At present additional minor changes in the diets are being made* so that the diagnosis of food sensitizations may be possible in a larger number of food sensitive patients.

THE FALLIBILITY OF SKIN TESTS

Ever since the first skin reactions were demonstrated to food and inhalant allergens over twenty-five years ago, it has been hoped that the various causes of allergy could be determined more conclusively and frequently by scratch or intradermal skin tests with improved and more stable allergens as they became available. *Increasingly,* however, *students of allergy have become convinced that clinical allergy may exist to inhalants and especially to foods in the absence of positive skin tests.* The reacting bodies, which in the union with the specific allergens are responsible for the skin reactions and the patient's symptoms, are present in the cells of the tissues in which the symptoms originate and may be absent in the blood and the cells of the skin. Thus a patient's skin may fail to react to some or all of the foods which are producing clinical symptoms. Definite positive reactions with the scratch test may occur, especially to those foods which produce obvious symptoms within an hour or two after their ingestion, whereas negative reactions often occur to foods which produce symptoms several hours or one or two days after ingestion, or only after the foods have been eaten on two or more days in succession. Positive reactions may also be obtained by the scratch and intradermal methods to foods productive of mild or delayed symptoms. *When positive skin reactions are associated with actual symptoms, the degree of clinical allergy in general cannot be determined by the size of such skin tests,* especially with the intradermal tests. Thus, diets

(13)

excluding only the foods giving the largest reactions are unscientific and practically always futile. Finally, it must be stressed that *many positive reactions, unfortunately, are not associated with clinical allergy*, but are indicative of past or potential allergy not affecting the patient, or are due to an irritable skin, or to toxic or non-specific substances in the allergens used for the tests.

TEST NEGATIVE DIETS

In spite of the vagaries of skin testing for food allergy, *certain patients are relieved by diets eliminating skin reacting foods.* Such diets excluding reacting foods have been well named *Test Negative Diets. This relief of a few patients unfortunately has encouraged many physicians to place unwarranted dependence on the test negative diets.* As stated above, the exclusion of the foods giving the largest skin reactions, especially by the intradermal method, nearly always gives disappointing results. The fact that symptoms are not relieved by such diets, however, does not by any means exclude the possibility of food allergy as a cause of the symptoms. The actual allergenic effect of a suspected food, it must be stressed, can only be determined by the reproduction of the symptoms in the patient who has become symptom-free through the elimination of causative foods. Thus the Test Negative Diets frequently exclude foods not productive of allergy. This is especially true if the intradermal test is used, since it often gives false reactions or those indicative of past or potential sensitization. Some allergists advise the exclusion of all foods which give even slight reactions by the intradermal tests. Retesting on several occasions is advised if relief does not occur. This may give additional reactions with a disappearance of others so that gradually most foods eaten by the patient may come under suspicion of possible allergy. This, of course, is accomplished at the outset of diet trial with the elimination diets but without the necessary use of intradermal testing which too often gives false reactions to foods or indicates potential or past allergy which has nothing to do with the patient's present symptomatology. Because of these facts, the intradermal test with food allergens has not been used by the writer as a routine for several years.

These test negative diets, moreover, often make the preparation of satisfactory meals quite difficult. Balanced meals with the essential protein, minerals, vitamins, and calories are often impossible to arrange with such non-reacting foods. Additional minerals and vitamins must also be prescribed by the physician to assure proper nutrition.

Thus, if test negative diets alone are used to diagnose food allergy, many patients will fail to receive relief and will be denied the benefit to be derived from the discovery and elimination of all allergenic foods. *These test negative diets are prescribed by the writer only when definite positive reactions obtained with the scratch test check with the patient's history of probable food idiosyncrasies.* In the large majority of his patients suspected of food allergy, however, the elimination diets, modified by the patient's history of probable food allergies and by definite skin reactions by the scratch method as described throughout this book are used for the diagnostic study of possible food allergy. *The elimination diets, moreover, may be used without the scratch tests if such are not available.*

MODIFIED ELIMINATION DIETS

When the elimination diets were first described, the writer suggested that physicians could modify them according to the patient's requirements in various countries or in various regions in our own country. Foods similar to those in the routine elimination diets might vary in availability and price. Thus Richet published slight modifications of the diets in France and various students have suggested varying changes in the elimination diets here in America. All of these contributions have added in different degrees to the availability and utility of trial diet and many menus and recipes have been evolved. *However, certain important aims for which the elimination diets originally were suggested have been lost sight of in some of these modifications.* The elimination diets intentionally, first of all, have contained as few foods which are infrequently productive of allergy as are required to prepare meals which can be taken for a period long enough for adequate study of the patient's possible food allergy. It would seem unwise therefore to add extra foods, spices, and beverages until the *object of diet trial has been attained—that is a symptom-free period which is definite and much longer than before diet trial was instituted.* Then with such a diet, productive of freedom from symptoms, various foods can gradually be added, leaving a period of five to seven days between each addition in order to determine thereby their allergenicity. *In the analysis of the allergenic effect of such additional foods, the varying time of the onset and degree of the reactivity of foods, the varying sites of tissue reaction of different foods, the variation in allergic tolerance itself, and the effect of natural desensitization or refractoriness which arises after or during an allergic reaction, must always be in mind.* These influences will be more fully discussed on page 56.

The fact that foods ingested over a long period of months or years may require omission from the diet for at least one or two weeks before evidence of clinical relief occurs is not fully appreciated by those who state that food allergy can be ruled out if symptoms are not relieved by the elimination of suspected foods for two or three days. In fact, the *persistent and chronic tissue changes arising from food and other allergies which are so evident in atopic eczema and also in chronic bronchial and nasal allergy, may require weeks or months of complete freedom from the causative allergens before cellular function and structure are restored.* Inhalant allergies may also necessitate weeks of hyposensitization or elimination before the tissues return to an approximately normal condition. Thus, it is necessary that elimination diets be so arranged that they can be eaten over a period of days, weeks, or even months without nutritional damage or undesirable weight loss as discussed on page 141.

The writer, moreover, has stressed the importance of the exclusion of every trace of food excluded from the elimination diets. Until the patient's symptoms are relieved and until a subtracted food can be fed to the symptom-free patient in order to actually determine the degree and severity of its clinical activity, it should be assumed that a maximum degree of allergy to that food exists. This is important since the sole object of the elimination diets is relief of symptoms. *Unfortunately some of the modified elimination diets proposed by others have included traces of foods which otherwise are excluded.* For instance, some have included butter or an oleomargarine. The latter contains varying minute amounts of milk which, however, are sufficient to prevent relief in patients markedly sensitive to milk. Even the odor of an allergenic food may produce symptoms in certain patients. Certain modifications of the elimination diets, moreover, have recommended Melba wheat toast or other heated denaturized foods such as canned milk. Here again, *clinical experience indicates that patients markedly sensitive to a given food cannot take such foods subjected to high temperatures.* Denaturization is not complete and clinical symptoms arise from their use even though sensitized guinea pigs will not react to such heated proteins. *These modified diets, moreover, at times have not provided the patient with explicit menus* and have not stressed the necessity of the elimination of every trace of a food not included in the actual diets. The rather frequent occurrence of pepper allergy is illustrative. Asthma in one patient and angioneurotic edema in another occurs if food containing a trace of pepper is eaten. Allergy to cottonseed was so great in another patient that the allergen in Crisco used in biscuits was enough to perpetuate asthma in the early morning hours. *Successful diet trial,* therefore,

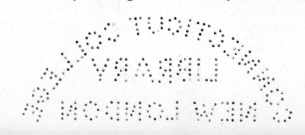

as will be noted throughout this book, *depends on the exclusion of every trace of a food not included in the prescribed diet and demands the meticulous preparation and supervision of meals, especially if eaten in friends' homes or in restaurants or hotels as discussed on page 176.* This care is absolutely necessary until relief from symptomatology occurs.

The elimination diets originally were formulated with these ideas in mind and my past and present modifications of them have insisted on the total exclusion of all foods not included in the diets. The proper preparation and arrangement of meals so that nutritional balance can be assured during a period long enough to rule food allergy in or out of the etiology are always necessary.

WHY ARE THE ELIMINATION DIETS PREFERABLE TO WHEAT-, MILK-, AND EGG–FREE DIETS?

Since wheat, milk, and eggs produce more allergy than any other three foods, physicians have frequently advised the exclusion of only these foods in trial diets. *Usually explicit menus and recipes for wheat-, milk-, and egg-free diets have not been given* so that small amounts of these foods unintentionally have been eaten. Since marked food allergy requires the complete exclusion of every trace of the allergenic foods, patients sensitive to these important foods, therefore, have not been relieved.

When the elimination diets with their menus as detailed in Chapter V are used, however, the patient is provided with positive directions of what he can eat, with recipes for bakery products which are wheat-, milk , and egg-free, and with balanced meals so that nutritional damage will not occur. *The elimination diets, therefore, provide the patient with accurate menus which are wheat-, milk-, and egg-free. Moreover, it must be remembered that much allergy also exists to other foods excluded from the elimination diets, especially to fish, nuts, spices, the cabbage group of vegetables, oranges, apples, bananas, berries, tea, coffee, honey, and other foods.* Thus, while wheat, milk, and eggs are being excluded, it is also wise to remember the frequency of allergy to the other foods just mentioned and to exclude them from the trial diet as has been done in the elimination diets. Allergy may also exist to the various foods in the elimination diets as discussed on page 145, but to a lesser degree than to those foods excluded from such diets. When allergy to foods in the diets is suspected or actually exists, other foods must be substituted as recommended in Chapter V. In a few patients with extensive food sensitizations, the supplemental diets outlined on page 181 may be necessary.

2

FOOD ADDITION DIETS

For one elimination diet, the writer has always recommended the sole use of milk for a period of one, two, or more weeks with the possible use of sugar and tapioca which rarely produce allergy. Such a diet may be used initially in infants, young children, and under-nourished adults who apparently have no idiosyncrasy to milk, who like it and digest it without difficulty. When possible allergy exists to it, the time devoted to its use in diet trial is often wasted, harmful, and nutritional and weight loss may occur. This diet, however, does control symptoms in patients who are sensitive to other foods than milk. Thereafter, every few days, individual foods, one or two at a time, may be added, excluding those which reproduce symptomatology.

The institution of diet trial with one food such as milk was especially advised by O. H. Brown who called such study *the food addition method.* Milk is the best food to use for this purpose since it can be taken together with its products such as cottage cheese, butter, and cream in amounts sufficient to maintain weight and nutrition over a period of two or more weeks or a shorter period if symptoms are thereby definitely controlled. *There are several disadvantages, however, in the milk diet.* Approximately 20 to 30 per cent of all food-sensitive patients seem allergic to milk in varying degrees. The probable mild or subclinical sensitizations to milk may be greater. Thus one out of every two or three patients may not be relieved by the milk diet after its sole use for two or three weeks.

Other diet trial with one food which will meet nutrition requirements is extremely difficult. If milk allergy is suspected and if maintenance of weight is not a problem, and if the patient's will power is adequate, peas, both fresh and in a split pea puree may be taken during the initial period. Other individual foods containing protein which will protect the protein metabolism such as meat or other legumes may also be used, providing undesirable weight loss does not result. Single foods other than milk for diet trial of seven to fourteen days, however, are difficult from the patient's view-point, and for necessary diet trial, the elimination diets are much more desirable and practicable. Confining the diet to milk for one or two weeks, moreover, is distasteful to most individuals and the sole use of any other food is much more difficult. *These objections are not present with the use of the elimination diets devoid of milk if they are properly prescribed and prepared as described in this volume.*

CHAPTER II

DIAGNOSIS OF ALLERGY

A careful analysis of the patient's history often yields information of great value in the final determination of possible allergenic causes. It is well recorded according to the outline found on page 216. The frequency of allergy as discussed on page 54 must be kept in mind in such history taking. Realizing that allergy may arise from substances entering the body through the mouth and digestive tract, inhaled and absorbed through the nasopharynx, conjunctivæ and the bronchial tract, entering the tissues from foci of infection or from diseased tissue in the body itself or from contact with skin, the patient must be questioned by the physician with all these possible types of allergy in mind.

ALLERGIC HISTORY

Allergy should be suspected if any of the recognized manifestations of allergy are present in the past or present history of the patient or have occurred in the family history, especially in the parents, aunts, uncles, grandparents, and even in the cousins.

Summary of Manifestations.—These manifestations of allergy which are more fully discussed in Chapter IV follow. *Since allergy may affect any tissue in the body it is obvious that many other results of allergy may exist than those summarized below.*

1. *Nasal allergy or hay fever*, seasonal or perennial, characterized by nasal congestion or blocking, watery or mucoid discharge, sneezing, tickling or itching of the nose, pharynx, palate, or Eustachian tubes; repeated so-called "head colds" with or without fever or recurrent so-called sinusitis without fever.

2. *Bronchial asthma, recurrent bronchitis*, or long-continued irritative dry coughs with or without wheezing, especially with exercise or in the early morning hours.

3. *Urticaria (hives) or recurring swellings* (angioneurotic edema) in the skin of various parts of the body or in the mouth, tongue, or throat; *dermatitis or eczema*, characterized by itching, erythema, dryness, scaling, thickening, or cracking of varying areas and amounts of the skin; *acneform eruptions* due to allergy.

4. *Ocular congestion, redness, itching*, with watery or mucoid discharge; recurring corneal ulcers.

5. *Disturbances in the mouth, pharynx, and gastro-intestinal tracts*, including cracking and dermatitis of the lips, corners of the mouth,

(19)

and on the skin around the mouth, recurrent "cold sores" on the lips, canker sores, redness, soreness, raw or white patches on the membrane of the cheeks, gums, tongue, palate or pharynx; fullness or swelling in the esophagus; distention, fullness in the upper and middle abdomen; soreness, belching, anorexia, nausea, vomiting indicative of possible allergy in the stomach; soreness, distention cramping in the lower abdomen; diarrhea, constipation, mucus in the bowel movement; recurrent or constant so-called ulcer or appendiceal pain in the absence of definite pathology; pain or spasm in the rectum, and finally mild or severe itching (pruritus) of the anus.

6. *Recurrent headaches or migraine* with or without nausea, vomiting or abdominal pain often associated with half blurred vision, colored or scintillating lights before the eyes, disturbances in smell, hearing, taste, or in the sensations throughout the body or with transient weakness or even paralysis of the musculature of the body.

7. *Painful, burning, or frequent urination or pain* suggestive of kidney or ureteral colic without pathological findings in the urine or the urological tract; *painful or abnormal menstruation or leucorrhea* not associated with gynecological or endocrine abnormalities.

8. *Painful, red, swollen, and at times enlarged, stiffened joints*, especially recurrent swelling with fluid in one or several joints.

9. Certain irregularities and other disturbances in the *heart* and the *vascular tissues* further discussed on page 138.

10. Allergic purpura, allergic toxemia characterized by fatigue, drowsiness and mental confusion, and allergic fever due to food, drug and at times to other sensitizations.

It must be stressed as it is in Chapter IV that allergy is responsible for this long list and variety of symptoms in varying degrees of frequency and that *allergy is only one of their several causes that needs careful consideration by the physician.* Allergy needs more definite study when certain manifestations such as asthma, hay fever, eczema, or migraine are present than when nausea, constipation, or menstrual disturbances occur. However, the *physician must keep allergy in mind as a possible factor in the problem of all patients seen*, as is indicated by the discussion of allergy in the average population on page 54. Such adequate study of the allergic possibilities is especially necessary when any of the symptoms listed above are present.

Family History of Allergy.—*The importance of a carefully recorded family history of possible allergy as a diagnostic aid needs emphasis.* Though all persons are victims of one or another type of allergy as noted on page 54, the propensity to develop allergy and the *degree and type of allergic manifestations are definitely heightened and influenced by heredity*. Allergy in both sides of the family predisposes to more definite allergy in the progeny than when it is present in one parent or his relatives. Analysis of family histories reveals the tendency for one manifestation such as asthma, nasal allergy, dermatitis or migraine to occur in a number of relatives. This, however, does not exclude the occurrence of other manifestations. Many patients may have several manifestations simultaneously, one being of special severity. Moreover, the tendency to develop pollen, animal emanation, or food allergy frequently is determined by inheritance and the susceptibility to allergy to one food such as milk, egg, fish, or fruit occasionally may run through the members of several generations.

Diet History.—*A dietary history must be carefully recorded in every patient suspected of allergy.* It would seem a wise routine in all patients seen by any physician since food sensitizations, at times of great importance, thereby can often be appreciated. The physician should first of all ask, "Are there any foods you definitely dislike or that disagree with you?" An affirmative answer may occur, in which case, more details about reactions to such foods should be obtained. Then specific questions about each food should be asked. "Do you drink milk?" Frequently the answer will be, "I hate milk," or "I never took it willingly since infancy," or "It always nauseates me," or "It is poison to me." Other specific questions such as "Do you eat eggs?" if not "Why don't you?" "Do you like and eat meat?" should be asked. Similar questions about fish, nuts, vegetables, fruit, bread and bakery products yield information which will justify the expended time. Habits of eating, whether or not symptoms occur after banquets, meals at restaurants or in friends' homes must be questioned so that unusual foods causing allergy may be found. The diagnostic value of a history of food dislikes and disagreements is discussed on page 58.

Drug Allergies.—*A history of possible drug allergies should be routine* in the study of all allergic patients. The drugs which most frequently produce allergy are noted on page 99. Direct questions such as "Does aspirin agree with you?" "Has quinine, if taken, upset you?" "What physics do you take?" "Is phenolphthalein in any of them?" "Does codein or morphine cause nausea or other distress?" "What other medicines have been taken and have any disagreed?" "What ointments, salves, hair lotions, dentifrices, mouth washes, douching solutions are used?" "Do they cause any irritation, burning or eruptions?" These and other questions must be asked to assemble all such information for analysis.

Causes of inhalant and contactant allergies as discussed in Chapter III *can often be suspected from a carefully taken history.* Careful analysis of the patient's daily and weekly routine may suggest such an allergen encountered only in the house, office, on the train, in a friend's home, during recreation, or in some other special environment. Allergy to causes such as cat, horse, or other animal hair, feed or grain dusts, species of fungi encountered in damp houses, orris root, or karaya gum at the hair dresser's, various plant or pollen allergens in gardens or open country may thus be found.

Environmental History.—*The so-called environmental history is an important part of all histories* of allergic patients. The trees, shrubs, flowers, vegetation, animals, fowl, and even vines on the house encountered around the home or during the daily routine should be noted. If on a farm, the type of work done, the kind of hay, feed, and farm products exposed to is important.

In the house, the number in the family, the type of work each performs, whether the dust from work or recreation is brought into the home, kind of mattresses, bedding, pillows, carpets, animals or birds in the house, animal skins, furs, insect powders or chemicals in the rooms or closets, and other similar questions will reveal information at times of great value. When contact dermatitis is suspected, the substances touching the skin, or oils or resins as from poison ivy or other vegetation which, air borne, might deposit on the skin must be carefully studied as possible causes.

The history of the patient, as discussed above, has long been taken and assembled by the writer according to the plan as presented on page 216. Following such a routine is a great aid to the physician since it assures thoroughness of analysis and the grouping of information.

As a definite aid in obtaining important information from the patient, a questionnaire as presented on page 209 is offered. This can be filled out by the patient during his absence from the office and with the help of the family. The answers may be very helpful to the physician for diagnosis of possible allergy.

SKIN TESTING

Cause and Mechanism of Reactions.—When the allergen or reacting substance of foods, inhalants, certain drugs, and bacteria comes in intimate contact with the cells of the skin just below the superficial epidermal surface, a skin reaction may occur. *The reaction depends on the presence of so-called reacting bodies in these cells of the patient who is specifically allergic or hypersensitive to the allergen of the substance being tested. These reacting bodies, however, may not be present in the cells of the skin or blood and may only occur in the cells of the shock tissue wherein arise the allergic symptoms.* The negative skin reaction in the presence of active allergy to an allergen is thereby explained as already discussed on page 13. *The positive reaction arises from increased permeability of the capillaries in the affected skin area* with resultant edema or accumulation of plasma, lymph, white, and eosinophilic blood cells in the tissue. Vascular dilatation, producing erythema, may surround the edematous hive-like swelling or wheal. The edema may follow the peripheral lymph channels producing "out-pushing" or pseudopodia and consequent irregularities in the outline of the wheal. The reaction occurs within ten to twenty minutes, its speed of appearance and its size depending on the number of reacting bodies in the skin, and usually on the degree of allergy present. However, *at times, large skin reactions may only indicate potential allergy and be unaccompanied by clinical manifestations.* The reaction begins to fade in twenty to forty minutes and may be entirely absent in one or two hours. However, in patients with large reactions and especially marked allergy, deep cutaneous and even subcutaneous edema may occur, persisting for one or two days. So-called delayed reactions may arise in six, twelve, or twenty-four hours after the test. These consist of a red papule $\frac{1}{8}$ to $\frac{1}{4}$ inch in diameter which may be surrounded by erythema and exude a small amount of purulent or serous exudate.

Scratch or Puncture Test.—*All skin testing should first be done by the scratch or puncture test. Intradermal tests should only be done with allergens which have failed to react by the scratch technic* since the initial intradermal testing has led to severe and dangerous constitutional reactions when done with allergens which would give positive scratch tests. The scratch test is executed by making a superficial scratch $\frac{1}{4}$ inch long with a dull knife or needle so that blood is not drawn. The allergen is then applied with toothpick or dropper. If a dry allergen is used, it is best moistened with N/10 NaOH or with normal salt solution. The allergen is then rubbed into the scratch with a clean toothpick. *The so-called puncture test may replace the scratch test in the future.* It is done by piercing the skin with a sterile needle through a drop of applied liquid allergen. The tests are best made on the upper arms, forearms and back, though the legs and abdomen may be used, especially if patients do not wish the scratches to show. *Under no circum-*

stances can 10 per cent NaOH be substituted for the dilute N/10 NaOH.
Necrosis of the skin and permanent scarring will result if the former strength is used. The patients, other than infants and small
children, can be tested with 180 to 250 food, animal emanations,
dust, and inhalant allergens and all important pollens on the arms
and back by experienced technicians in two to three hours. It may
be best to do such testing in two different sittings. Infants and
young children should be tested on several occasions only with
the most important foods and ingestants, reserving the less important ones for future testing if symptoms are not adequately relieved
by treatment:

Intradermal Test.—*Intradermal tests are done only with those
allergens which fail to react by the scratch test.* When the extracts
are standardized by nitrogen determinations, an extract containing 0.01 mg. per cc. may be initially injected. In the presence of
a negative test, a stronger extract may be used later if desired.
In the writer's work, 1 to 200 dilutions of the dry allergens are
routinely used for intradermal testing. Later, a 1 to 50 glucose
extract may be used if negative reactions with the 1 to 200 extracts
have occurred. The intradermal injection of a concentrated
glycerin extract, however, will produce a localized necrosis. The
amount injected intracutaneously should be between 0.01 and
0.02 cc. The resultant reaction has characteristics similar to the
positive scratch test. From 10 to 60 of these intradermal tests
may be done at one time on the patient other than the infant or
young child without fear of constitutional reactions, providing no
allergen which has reacted by the scratch method is used. *With
this precaution, it is possible to test a patient by the scratch and intradermal methods in one or two days and also obtain the necessary
history, physical examination, laboratory, and x-ray studies in the
same period.* This conserves the patient's time and is an economic
saving to him.

*In the writer's practice, intradermal tests are done with all impor-
tant inhalant allergens which have not reacted by the scratch method.
Routine intradermal testing with food allergens which have not reacted
by the scratch test is not done, since many confusing, false, and certain
negative reactions occur as previously discussed on page* 13. Elimination diets are depended upon in the majority of patients, rather
than the test negative diets, as formerly noted on page 14.

Passive Transfer (Prausnitz and Küstner) Test.—*The passive transfer reaction is utilized occasionally* in patients who are so
young, so sick or so covered with dermatitis that skin testing is
inadvisable or impossible. Prausnitz and Küstner, in 1921, dis-

covered that the serum of a patient clinically sensitive to a food to which a large skin reaction occurs, contains skin reacting bodies. If small amounts of this serum are injected into many different areas of the skin of normal people, these areas may be tested with ingestant and inhalant allergens in twenty-four or more hours. Reacting bodies to specific allergens present in the serum of the patient can thereby be demonstrated in the skin of the recipient. He must be a person who gives a positive reaction with injected serum containing reacting bodies to a known allergen. False positive and also negative reactions occur and the results of the testing must perforce be checked by clinical trial or confirmed by the therapeutic test. This method of testing requires careful laboratory technic, and must be reserved for specialists' use in occasional, selected cases.

Ocular and Nasal Tests.—*Since inhalant allergens give negative skin reactions in 10 to 20 per cent of patients clinically sensitive to such allergens,* and since the nasobronchial and ocular mucous membranes frequently harbor reacting bodies not present in the skin, the dry or liquid extracts of various inhalants, especially pollens, may be deposited on the conjunctival sac, applied or blown into one nostril, or blown or sprayed into the bronchial tract. Ocular redness and congestion, symptoms of nasal allergy or of bronchial asthma, according to the site of application, within five to thirty minutes are indicative of specific allergy to the allergen used. *This ocular or nasal test* at times is also used to determine the clinical activity of various pollens or other inhalants that have given positive skin reactions.

ALLERGENS AND THEIR PREPARATION

The active substance in inhaled or ingested substances to which a patient becomes sensitized is called an *allergen*. When allergy is established, so-called *reacting bodies* develop in the body, attaching themselves especially to the cells of the tissues in which the major reactivity arises which is responsible for the patient's symptoms. These reacting bodies are comparable, but probably not identical to the immune or antibodies and precipitins of immunity. They are present to a greater or less degree in the cells of the entire body, and, in the markedly sensitive patients, are present in the blood, as demonstrable by the Prausnitz-Küstner reaction, and in the skin, as evidenced by positive skin reactions. These allergens are either protein in nature or apparently need conjugation with protein to produce sensitization. Some evi-

dence indicates that a carbohydrate, at times, is primarily responsible, requiring, however, union with a body protein to create the
specific allergy. *Such union of body protein with simple or complex chemicals* such as chlorine, arsenic, mercury, dyes, aspirin,
sulfanilamide, and many other chemicals used in industry and
medicine which may contact or enter the body, explains why
allergy develops to such chemicals in so many people. Such substances, which in union with a body protein determine the specificity of the resultant allergic reactivity, are called "*haptens.*"

Skin reactions in sensitized patients can be obtained with actual
foods, animal emanations, dusts, or other inhaled substances and
at times with drugs. Thus, dry pollens, finely pulverized animal
emanations, orris root, pyrethrum, cottonseed, kapok, or the
ground dried foods may be used for testing. The fresh uncooked
foods give reactions in many sensitized patients. *In order to
preserve these allergens, however, and to obtain a concentrated preparation of them,* various technics have been evolved by which dry
powders containing the specific proteins or reacting substances,
are prepared or fluid extracts are made. The technic of their
preparation is described in current textbooks. (See page 257.)
Much work has been done to obtain allergens in powdered or
liquid form which are stable over long periods of time, which give
good reactions on the skins of patients known to be clinically
sensitive to the allergens, and in getting as high a concentration
of the reacting substances in the so-called allergen as possible.
The fluid extracts of inhalants and foods at present are usually
prepared with glycerin or glucose extracting fluids to which but-
tered salt solution and a weak preservative are added. Though
the glycerin extracts may maintain their activity a little longer
than the glucose extracts, the latter have the advantage of not
causing false reactions during skin testing. *The activity and
potency of allergens used for skin testing must be assured by their
production of positive reactions in the skins of patients known to be
clinically sensitive to the allergens in question.* Allergens should be
checked every few months since deterioration at times occurs,
especially in fluid extracts made with salt solution.

How Much Skin Testing is Indicated?—*Even though skin
reactions to inhalants, and especially to foods, may be negative when
clinical sensitization is present, and though non-specific or positive
reactions in the absence of clinical allergy occur, especially by the
intradermal test, routine skin testing of patients suspected of allergy
is most important.* Food allergy, as already stated, which produces definite or immediate symptoms, usually is indicated by

good scratch reactions. More delayed, cumulative, or chronic symptoms from food allergy are frequently associated with negative scratch and less often with negative intradermal tests. Inhalant sensitizations more often are associated with positive scratch, and especially positive intradermal reactions, though negative tests or indefinite reactions occur by both methods, as already discussed on page 24. In spite of the fact, however, that the skin test does not yield final information, careful testing with all important foods, animal emanations, a considerable number of miscellaneous inhalants, house dust, spores of important fungi, and important spring, summer, fall, cultivated flower and tree pollens as discussed in Chapter III should be routine in most patients.

Patients suspected of food allergy alone should be tested with all important food allergens and with a moderate number of inhalant allergens of all types. If reactions to such inhalants occur, indicative of unsuspected sensitizations, then complete testing with inhalants by the scratch and checked by intradermal testing would be desirable.

It must be remembered that *the clinical significance of all positive reactions can only be assured by the production of actual symptoms in the patient by the ingestion or inhalation of the allergenic substance in question.*

Moreover, when skin testing is not available, many problems of food allergy can be worked out by information obtained from a well-taken history and the use of elimination diets as detailed in Chapter V.

Symptoms suggestive of, and usually due to food allergy are, at times, due to inhalant allergy as illustrated recently by a patient relieved of migraine by elimination diets who later developed severe upper left abdominal pain, found to be due to pollen allergy alone. Migraine or recurrent headaches, moreover, which are usually due to food allergy, at times are due to inhalant allergy with or without food sensitization as a cause. Skin testing with group allergens containing the group *allergens of closely related foods* is not advisable since mild reactions to one or two such allergens in the mixture used for testing may be missed.

Patients suspected of inhalant allergy should be routinely tested with food and inhalant allergens. Such complete testing is especially necessary in these individuals since uncontrolled food, animal emanation, or miscellaneous allergen allergy in a pollen sensitive patient, for example, will often prevent good results from pollen hyposensitization therapy. This routine and complete testing is not difficult in experienced hands, and when scratch testing as described on page 23 is followed by intradermal tests with those important allergens which have failed to react by the scratch test, such skin testing with between 200 and 300 allergens can be completed in two to three hours according to the speed of the technician. Emphasis must be laid on the fact that positive reactions must check with the clinical history or be confirmed by the reproduction of symptoms either by the ingestion or inhalation of the allergen in question during a symptom-free period. History, moreover, often indicates the causative allergy in the absence of skin reactivity.

Patch Tests in Contact Allergy.—The characteristics and nature of contact allergy and the use of patch testing in the diagnosis of it are discussed on page 100.

Diet and Daily Diaries.—The careful recording by the patient of all foods eaten and of various symptoms experienced during each day, at times, allows the physician or patient to discover specific foods which are responsible for certain manifestations of allergy. *The ability to discover foods, beverages, or condiments which in minute amounts cause allergy is restricted by such diet diaries unless the patient is eating at home, and unless every ingredient, including condiments, is listed.* Away from home, traces of milk, butter, wheat, egg, pepper, or spices, for example, may not be recognized in menus eaten by the patient, and thus they would not be included in such a daily record of ingested foods. Unless such diaries are accurate, the trouble incurred by their tabulation and the necessary time spent by the physician in their analysis, are hardly justified. A suggested form for the keeping of a diary will be found on page 221.

The writer does not ask patients to prepare diet diaries because of the fallibility of such reports. It has been found that insistence on the strict limitation of the diet only to those foods included in the elimination diet prescribed for the patient allows a more accurate analysis of the effects of such foods than results from diet diaries described above. When an elimination diet is being taken, *the physician must interview the patient one to two times a week* to be certain that no trace of any food not prescribed is being taken. *The care with which foods are prepared* in the home kitchen must be questioned. Unwittingly or intentionally, the cook or patient may be including a little forbidden milk, butter, wheat, or other cereal flour, pepper, spice, or other food. *The fact that a trace of a food to which marked sensitization exists may prevent the clearing of resultant symptoms, or may reproduce symptoms temporarily or* for an indefinite period if such amounts continue to enter the diet, even one or two times a week, must be emphasized to the patient. A taste of a causative food is justified in the patient's mind by his statement, "I thought that a little bit would not matter." With the milk-free diet, butter substitutes and oleomargarines, all of which contain more milk than does butter, must not be used. The use of canned milks, commercial and bakery foods such as malted milk, ovaltine, sausage, and other meat mixtures, must be forbidden, since all their ingredients are often impossible to ascertain. The analysis of foods taken in friends' homes and restaurants is even more important since without the most careful and intelligent ordering by the patient, small or even large amounts of foods not included in the elimination diet will be eaten. Such meals, however, can be obtained which contain only those foods prescribed for the patient if he orders or asks for specific foods as detailed on page 176. *Thus, rather than have a patient keep a diet diary, the writer has found that it is more helpful and profitable to devote his time to the careful analysis of the patient's meals at home and away therefrom, in order to be assured of the absolute accuracy of the patient's coöperation.*

A patient's diary of the various activities, routine of work, social and recreational engagements, with a record of various symptoms of possible allergic origin, is of considerable help at times in the determination of possible inhalant allergies. With such a diary, the physician can inquire about possible contacts with household allergens, animals in and out of doors, flowers, shrubs, trees, vines on the house, and other possible origins of inhalant allergens. When inhalant or contact allergies are suspected as causes of the patient's symptomatology, the physician must study the possibilities of all such allergens through careful questioning of the patient during conferences. Thus such a diary of activities as discussed above may be valuable in obscure or difficult problems.

The Determination of Allergenic Foods.—It has already been noted in Chapter I that most patients either fail to react to all foods to which allergy exists or give reactions which are nonspecific or which are not associated with any allergic manifestation. *When positive skin reactions are present, their rôle in the production of clinical allergy can only be determined by the feeding of the reacting foods to the symptom-free patient.* Definite exaggeration of symptoms or the recurrence of symptoms indicates probable allergy to the added food.

The unquestioned decision that a given food causes allergic reactivity is often difficult. Tolerance varies in every individual so that symptoms may recur immediately in a violent manner from a trace of food in some patients, or they may arise in a few hours or in two or three days, or the food may have to be taken for two or three weeks before symptoms recur.   The tendency for allergic manifestations to recur in cyclic attacks with periods of freedom due to desensitization or refractoriness has been noted on page 56. *To adequately study the effect of a suspected food, moreover, the patient should be freed from his allergic symptoms for a much longer period than has previously occurred before diet and other allergic therapy was instituted.*   The evidence indicating the allergenic foods, in many patients, is comparatively easy to obtain, especially if the patient gives a history of intolerance or idiosyncrasy to such foods.

Leucopenic Index.—A few years ago, Vaughan drew attention to the reduction in the white cell count in the blood after the ingestion of a markedly allergenic food.   This had been previously reported, especially by French observers, and Vaughan hoped that information might be obtained through white cell counts, before and after the ingestion of a given food, about its possible allergenicity. At present, *the routine use of this procedure in the study of possible food sensitizations has been discontinued*, since the necessary blood counts are time-consuming and fraught with too many possible and technical errors.   The reduction of the white cell count after the ingestion of foods to which definite allergy exists, however, is frequent and is often associated with an increase in the eosinophilic cells in the blood.

Eosinophilia and Other Changes in the Blood.—When active allergy to foods, inhalants, and at times, to bacteria, exists, the *granular, red staining, white blood cells (eosinophilic neutrophiles) are frequently increased.*   They usually rise from a normal of 1 to 2 per cent up to 4 to 10 per cent, though at times 25 to 50 per cent of the white blood cells are eosinophiles.   However, a normal count does not rule out allergy.   High eosinophilic counts are also found in diseases due to animal parasites and in the necrosing disease of the arteries called periarteritis nodosa. Such eosinophilia may be due to an allergic state in these diseases.

Eosinophilic cells are also abundant in the tissues which harbor the main allergic reactions.   Thus the bronchial and nasal mucosæ become infiltrated with eosinophiles in patients with bronchial asthma and perennial or seasonal hay fever.   The gastro-intestinal tissues and the skin contain an excess of such cells when they harbor localized allergy.   The secretions from such sensitized tissues, thus contain eosinophiles, the presence of which offers diagnostic evidence of allergy as noted on page 117.   Whether such eosinophilic cells are due to changes in the tissues themselves or have been attracted to such body tissues from the blood stream is not known.

The *total number of white blood cells is often increased in allergy*, especially in children and in attacks of bronchial asthma or gastro-intestinal allergy. The count may rise to 15,000 or 20,000. The polymorphonuclear cells are never as elevated as when such leuco-cytosis is due to pyogenic infections. Allergy and infection frequently exist together accounting for other changes in the leucocytic count.

Studies of the *calcium, phosphorus, potassium, and serum protein content of the blood* in allergic patients have failed to reveal any consistent abnormalities.

Diet Trial.—In the discovery of the various allergenic foods responsible for the allergic symptoms in the patient, *diet trial is of paramount value*. The fallibility of skin tests, the limited value to diet diaries, the impossibility of obtaining dependable information from the leucopenic index studies, and the limited help from careful dietary histories have all been discussed. With diet trial, however, the possibilities of food sensitizations can be best studied, especially if the elimination diets are utilized, as detailed in Chapter V, so that adequate diet trial, if necessary over a period of several weeks, becomes possible. With such elimination diets, sufficient time for such study can be taken since satisfying menus for regular meals are possible similar to those published herein and nutrition can be protected even with diet trial for long periods if the directions and precautions for the proper intake of proteins, minerals, vitamins, and calories, are followed. These elimination diets offer a practical method of studying possible food allergy and when modified and manipulated as described in this and former publications, the frequency of food allergy as a cause of its many manifestations as discussed in Chapter IV will be recognized. *The elimination diets must be used in the diagnostic study of patients in the same way that blood counts, urine analyses, or x-ray studies are used.* The use of any of these tests, of course, does not presuppose that the suspected disease such as food allergy, appendicitis, nephritis, or diabetes is present.

Environmental Control.—*When inhalant allergies* are indicated by history or by skin testing, the control of the environment in the home, working, or recreational areas, at times relieves the patient*

---

* For protection against dusts in various occupations there are many respirators which fit over nose and mouth. Tight goggles at times are advisable. The Willson Products, Inc., Reading, Pa., and the H. S. Cover, South Bend, Indiana, and especially the American Optical Co., San Francisco, Calif., make such respirators.

of his symptoms. Often hyposensitization, as described on page 40 is also necessary. When inhalant sensitizations are suspected, and a partial control of the environment and the indicated hyposensitization therapy do not produce desired relief, then the placing of the patient in a room in which strict control of the possible air-borne allergens is assured may be used as a diagnostic measure and for the control of symptoms. Therewith, hyposensitization can be given according to the resultant relief.

Strict environmental control can be established in the hospital or in most homes. Carpets must be removed from such a room, and washable throw rugs substituted. Ordinary wooden floors should be thoroughly washed and dried. Painting may be desirable. Hardwood floors or linoleum should be carefully cleaned. The fact that ingredients in paint, furniture polishes, and floor cleaners or waxes may cause or activate allergy in certain patients must be remembered. Overstuffed furniture in the room should be replaced by wooden, iron, or wicker without cushions. The mattress and pillows should be covered with slips made of thin, rubberized or lotus cloth,* best closed with zippers. Over such slips, several sheets, pillow slips, cotton pads, or towels should be placed to diminish the discomfort from sleeping on the non-absorbable rubberized material. A box spring may be encased with a rubberized slip or should be replaced by an open spring mattress. Bedding should be well-washed cotton or, if the patient is not wool sensitive, old, well-washed, woolen blankets, free of the fuzz of newness. No comforters (cotton, woolen, or feather) should be used since they throw off fine dust to which allergy may exist. Shades on the windows should be wiped free of dust. Draperies and curtains should be taken down, thoroughly washed or cleaned and simply rehung. Finally, the ceiling, walls, floors, woodwork, furniture, window frames, including the frame and springs of the bed, should be thoroughly wiped and cleaned with damp cloths to remove the dust and not brushed into the air. The floors and woodwork of such a room should be cleaned every day with damp cloths. Closets adjoining the room should be closed tightly or emptied of clothes and dust giving materials.

To prevent dust from adjoining rooms or halls from blowing into the patient's room, the doors must be closed and, preferably,

---

* A good rubberized cloth is made by Dupont. Lotus cloth is a light Chinese silk impregnated with rubber. It is sticky and gummy which may not be agreeable to the patient. The Expert Bedding Company of Chicago makes "Altex" encasings. The Allergen Products Company of Cleveland makes encasings from a Dupont rubberized fabric. Ready-made covers can be obtained from large department and mail order houses.

sealed with weather strips on door edges or with paper pasted thereon. All flowers, animals and perfumes and clothes should be kept out of the room. Friends and relatives should not remain long until good relief has occurred and no fur or woolen coats or dusty clothes should be worn in the room. Smoking and the use of cosmetics should be prohibited. As improvement occurs, the patient may use allergen-free cosmetics, though it should be realized that even these may secondarily initiate an underlying allergy or contain substances to which occasional allergy arises. At times, the cosmetics or clothing of nurses or relatives produce allergy in the patient. Silk sensitive patients may react to the allergens from silk stockings or clothing worn by nurses or friends. If the patient is pollen sensitive or lives in an area where much suspended dust is present in the air, an efficient pollen filter such as the improved one of the Carrier Corporation should be installed in the window to insure dust and pollen-free air in the room. This is especially important if the patient lives in the country where pollens are abundant or near barns or animal yards, especially when animal or feed dust allergy exists. Vines growing around the patient's windows, shrubs, and flowers in the garden near the room, birds roosting or nesting in the roof, or in vines or shrubs near the house, animal emanations, spores of molds and other dusts from adjoining roofs or yards may yield air-borne allergens which blow into the patient's room.

To study the effect of such an environmental control on presumed inhalant allergy, the patient should remain in such a room for a minimum of five days. If relief is evident, the diagnosis of inhalant allergy may be confirmed and further study and indicated therapy will gradually evidence the various etiological inhalant allergens and produce necessary hyposensitization. For a period of weeks or months, it may be necessary to spend varying amounts of time in such a room and to sleep therein. Because of this, a sitting room and, later, the patient's working environment or office may have to have a modified environmental control. Attention, also, may be necessary to the frequent cleaning of the automobile's interior, especially if animal emanations or house dust allergy is present.

THERAPEUTIC RESULTS IN DIAGNOSIS

The final determination of the various causes of allergic symptoms can only be arrived at after the results of the elimination of the allergens and hyposensitization with properly prepared extracts or antigens containing those allergens is ascertained. In food sensitive

3

patients, the initial object of study is to produce a symptom-free
period which is definitely longer than those which have previously
occurred.   When the patient or parents are certain that unquestioned relief has been established, the various foods can be added
at one- to two-week intervals as suggested in Chapter V and
gradually the foods responsible in varying degrees for the patient's
symptoms can be ascertained. Since hyposensitization or increased tolerance occurs with varying speed and frequency with
such elimination of foods, at times the reinstatement of a formerly
allergenic food in the diet is not associated with symptoms, though
they may arise at a later date as discussed on page 59.   Likewise,
the causes of inhalant, contactant, and the less frequent bacterial
allergies must gradually be determined through the careful analysis
of protection against such allergens and subsequent exposure to
them when the patient is symptom-free, and especially through
the results of hyposensitization with antigens containing those
allergens which cannot be removed from the patient's everyday
environment.   *Thus the absolute determination of all of the allergenic
causes of many allergic manifestations requires intelligent and understanding coöperation and analysis of the patient and the evaluation
of well-directed and adequate therapy by the physician, at times over
a period of months or even several years.*   Relief which is adequate
or nearly complete may occur in a brief period of days or weeks,
but the unequivocable decision as to number and degree of activity
of all the causative allergens, many of them possibly producing a
mild or so-called subclinical effect, may be extremely difficult.
With all these ideas in mind, therefore, it is seen, that diagnosis of
the allergenic causes depends, as does all medical diagnosis in a
varying degree, on the results of therapy.

CHAPTER III

CAUSES OF ALLERGY AND THEIR CONTROL

Allergy may arise to any substance with which the body tissues have contact either through ingestion, inhalation, actual contact through the skin, absorption from foci of infection or acute infections, absorption from products from diseased tissues, or from medicaments given for therapeutic reasons. Allergy due to ingested, inhaled, or injected substances or from foci of infection or diseased tissues is due to allergens which enter the blood and which are carried by the blood all over the body. They are hematogenously borne allergens. Such allergens sensitize every cell in the body in varying degrees. *Those tissues which have a predisposition to develop allergy either through some natural cause and especially through inheritance are more highly sensitized than others and when the substance is ingested, inhaled, or absorbed thereafter, the allergic reaction in such tissues is so great that cellular changes arise which produce symptoms.* Thus patients may have one or more of the ordinary or less common manifestations of allergy such as bronchial asthma, hay fever, perennial nasal allergy, eczema, urticaria, migraine or gastro-intestinal symptoms described in Chapter IV according to the localization of the reacting bodies sufficient in degree to produce tissue disturbances. It may well be that the cells of the blood-vessels and especially of the capillaries are primarily sensitized when allergy develops, and that sensitization of the surrounding tissue cells develops thereafter. *That every cell in the body is sensitized more or less is evidenced in a patient suffering with hay fever or asthma who develops a so-called general reaction* when an excessive dose of the allergen is injected. The explanation of such reactions is given on page 42. *Contact allergy contrasted with the types discussed above is dependent on reacting bodies in the superficial skin cells and possibly in mucous membranes. This will receive further consideration on page 99.*

The various allergens which are known to produce clinical symptoms are grouped in the following tabulation. They will be discussed in the remainder of this chapter.

1. *Inhalants*

Pollens	Hay and feed dusts
Animal and bird emanations	House dusts
	Occupational dusts
Silk	Recreational dusts

1. *Inhalants (Continued)*

Orris root
Cosmetics
Pyrethrum
Flaxseed
Kapok
Cottonseed
Glue

Flours and dusts from other
  foods
Drugs and medicaments
Fly and insect emanations
Spores of fungi and smuts
Tobacco
Chemical inhalants

2. *Ingestants*

Foods
Beverages
Condiments

Drugs
Water (mineral and
  organic contents)

3. *Contactants*

Environmental
Medicinal

Occupational
Cosmetic

4. *Infectants including bacteria, parasites and fungi.   Products of diseased tissues*

5. *Insect and snake bites*

6. *Injectants*

(*a*) Subcutaneous or intramuscular

Sera
Drugs
Hormones
Allergens

Vaccines
Snake and bee venom
Catgut

(*b*) Intravenous

Sera
Drugs
Allergens

Vaccines
Foods (through transfu-
  sion)

(*c*) Rectally

Drugs

Foods

(*d*) Nasal, aural sinus, vaginal, urological, intrabron-
chial, cerebrospinal injections of drugs, sera or
allergens

7. *Physical allergy*

Either primary or secondary in action

INHALANT ALLERGENS

Pollens. — *Pollens are the most common inhalants to cause allergy.*
They most frequently produce seasonal nasal allergy or hay fever,
seasonal and at times chronic bronchitis or bronchial asthma,

seasonal ocular allergy and atopic dermatitis or eczema. Recurrent headache or migraine and gastro-intestinal symptoms may also arise from pollen allergy. Being the germinal and vital elements of the flower and rich in protein, pollens readily produce sensitization.

The morphology or shape of distantly related pollens is dissimilar. Each pollen is quite constant in size and shape and closely related species are nearly identical. The features and characteristics of pollens have been studied especially by Wodehouse. Those of a number of important pollens are given in Table 1. Pollen grains have definite morphology, those of closely related species and genuses being similar, their size varying from 6 to 12 μ ($\frac{1}{1000}$ cm.).

Table 1.—Morphology of Certain Allergy–producing Pollen Grains

	Shape	Type	Average size (μ)
I. Shrubs, grasses and weeds:			
A. Echinate	1. Spherical	Ambrosia	16–25
(Probably all Compositæ		Franseria	18–23
except Artemisia)		Xanthium	22–29
		Iva	25
		Helianthus	38
	2. Ellipsoidal	Hemizonia	38–29
B. Smooth	1. Ellipsoidal	Artemisia	18–28
	(Polyhedric)	Urticaceæ	12–25
		Ricinus	33–46
	2. Spherical	Plantago	34
	3. Polyhedric	Gramineæ	28–55
C. Punctate, with furrows .	. . . .	Brassica	25–46
D. With bands	1. Ellipsoidal	Rumex	22–32
E. With distinct pores . .	1. Spherical	Amaranthus	23–30
F. With less distinct pores .	1. Spherical	Atriplex	29
		Chenopodium	29
		Salicornia	29
G. Four grains held together .	. . . .	Typhaceæ	18–26
II. Trees:			
A. Punctate	1. Spherical	Populus	29
	2. Ellipsoidal	Garryaceæ	38
B. Three-lobed	1. Smooth		
	a. Blunt ends	Fagaceæ	25–40
		Plantanaceæ	17–25
		Oleaceæ	21–33
	b. Less blunt	Aceraceæ	28–36
	c. Pointed ends	Palmaceæ	13–25
	(one groove)		
	2. Punctate	Salix	18–29
C. Hemispherical	. . . .	Juglandaceæ	30–48
D. Two-winged	1. Reticulate	Pinaceæ	45–65
E. Polyhedric	1. Smooth	Betulaceæ	20–40
		Cupressaceæ	32
F. Triangular	1. Smooth	Eucalyptus	25
G. Gridiron	1. Spherical	Acacia	48–55

Pollens from inconspicuous wind pollinated flowers are so light that they are wafted into the air and remain there for long periods, being blown for many miles, finally being washed out of the air along with other matter by long and generalized storms. Such pollens along with spores of fungi, smuts, and bacteriæ are found in the air at an elevation of 15,000 feet or higher and Lindbergh even found them in the air over the Greenland ice cap. *Pollens may be counted in the air* by determining microscopically the number on 1 sq. cm. of a glass slide covered with a thin layer of vaseline or glycerin jelly, which slide has been exposed out of doors for a twenty-four-hour period. Knowing the morphological characteristics of the pollens as indicated in Table 1, the pollens can be counted and identified. Pollen counts vary in every area, not only in regard to the variety, but also the numbers. After the frosts, and especially with snow on the ground, the pollen rapidly disappears from the air. In the spring to fall months, rain temporarily reduces or eliminates the pollens, though the moisture, especially with subsequent warm days, is conducive to more and abundant pollination. In California, whenever sun and no rain are present, pollen is in the air. Tree pollens are most abundant from February to May, grass pollens from April to July and the amaranth, atriplex, ambrosia, Russian thistle, artemisia, and franseria pollens from July to November. Maximum pollen counts in California are not much greater than 400 to 500, being less in the cities than in the country, and especially in cities near the bay or ocean. In the Middle West and East where ragweed is the main fall pollen, counts may rise to 4000 or more. Allergists are able with frequent pollen counts or with counts on air near the patient's home to determine the predominant pollens or some specific environmental pollens which need special consideration in therapy.

Pollens of insect pollinated trees, shrubs, and flowers are not as important causes of allergy as are the wind borne pollens. However, patients may become sensitized to any of them especially if they live in close proximity. Flowers, shrubs, and trees around or on the house or in nearby yards may throw pollens which are blown for 50 or even 200 feet. Patients in the yards, in the street, or in the house may thus inhale those pollens. Blossoms and flowers in the house may also be responsible for allergic reactivity. Thus patients should also be skin tested with all important insect-borne pollens to which they are exposed.

A knowledge of the pollens which are in the air of the patient's environment is essential for successful therapy. With the aid of botanists, *surveys of most areas of the United States* and of certain other areas of the world have been made which include all of the pollen producing grasses, weeds, trees, shrubs, and flowers which are of importance in each area. Such surveys and abbreviated lists are available in the literature and in the larger texts for most areas of this country. The physician not only must know the flora of the immediate area, but that of distant areas, even 200 or more miles away, from which pollen carrying winds blow toward the patient's resident region. A knowledge of the shrubs, flowers, and trees around the patient's home is also very necessary in many cases. Since the pollens, and as we will later learn, the spores of fungi from various grain and farm products grown in farming areas around a country home, may produce marked and specific allergy, the physician's inquiry and survey should list all such possible causes. It is also important to remember that pollens in the air during the seasons may settle on the walls, curtains and carpets so that the *house dust may contain enough pollen to keep pollen allergy active through the winter months.*

Pollens are gathered by specially trained workers from the blooms of the grasses, shrubs, weeds, trees, and cultivated flowers themselves. The blooms just as they are about to yield pollen are collected in large numbers. The stems may be placed in low jars containing water so that the blooms hang over large sheets of glass or glazed paper, being in a draftless, light, preferably sunny and warm room. As the blossoms develop, pollen matures and either falls or is shaken on to the glass or paper. Then with a small camel-hair brush or razor blade the pollen is gathered. Those blooms which contain abundant pollen such as those of the artemisias and ambrosias may be pounded or rolled in the dried state. Pollen and dust obtained is then passed through a fine sieve several times to get as pure pollen as possible. It usually must be cleaned by passing through a 200 mesh screen. It is then dried over calcium chloride, defatted with ether, and stored in air-tight bottles. The allergist should have pollens available to test patients from nearby as well as distant areas, for which he often has 250 to 350 pollens of all types.

Evidence is increasing that there are active substances discussed on page 62 which are specific for each pollen. Closely related species such as grasses probably *contain allergens common to all grasses and also species-specific allergens found only in the single grass pollen. Such group and species-specific allergens are found in other closely related pollens such as the artemisia, ambrosia, franseria, or chenopod pollens.* This specificity of pollen allergens, therefore, demands that the physician know the various species of the grasses, weeds, trees, and flowers in the environment of the patient and that extracts of the pollen of such species be included in the antigens for the patient's treatment if the best results are to be obtained.

Method of Extraction.—*Pollens are extracted with solutions of* weak alkali or sodium chloride containing 35 to 50 per cent glycerin or with a 5 per cent glucose solution to which 4 per cent phenol has been added. Those extracts made with salt solution alone are not as stable. Usually 2 or 3 per cent extracts of the pollens are prepared, though some allergists maintain that all the active substance is extracted when 5 per cent or even 10 per cent preparations are made. The physician may include 10 or even 30 different pollen extracts in one bottle or may prepare several bottles of antigen for each patient, each containing 1 to 5 pollen extracts. *The amount of each pollen extract depends on the importance of that pollen in the patient's problem as determined by history skin testing, and the abundance of the pollen in the patient's territory.* If a 2 per cent stock extract of pollens is used, this 1 to 50 preparation is diluted to 1 to 500 and 1 to 5000 strengths. In very sensitive patients, initial treatment may require a 1 to 50,000 or a 1 to 500,000 or even a more dilute extract. When the antigen contains 10 or more pollens, a stronger dilution can be given originally than when it contains only 1 to 5 pollens. The maximum dose of an antigen with many pollens must be greater than when it contains a few.

Pollen Units.—The *usual unit of pollen allergen is the so-called Noon unit,* 1 unit being the amount of allergen in $\frac{1}{1000000}$ gram of dry pollen. Various students have standardized pollen extracts by total nitrogen or total protein nitrogen determinations. Equivalent amounts of these different preparations are given on page 226. Generally, it is conceded that standardization of pollen extracts by weight is best for therapeutic purposes.

Treatment.—*Treatment must be started with 0.05 or 0.1 cc. of a dilution which fails to react by the scratch test and especially which does not produce or exaggerate clinical symptoms.* It is rarely possible to start with a less dilute extract than a 1 to 5000 dilution, and often a 1 to 50,000 or even a 1 to 50,000,000 dilution must be used. Such weak extracts are especially necessary if only one or two pollens are combined in the antigen bottle and if the patient is extremely sensitive and if treatment is being given during the season. At such times, the amount of pollen in the air plus that which is injected may exceed the patient's tolerance and give rise to increased clinical symptoms. *At no time during therapy should symptoms be increased or reëstablished by pollen therapy.* Routine directions and fast and slow schedules for pollen administration are on page 218.

Three plans of pollen therapy are available: 1. *The pre-seasonal therapy* may be started three or four months before the pollen season begins. The treatments may be given every one to three days and a maximum dose of 0.60 to 1 cc. may finally be reached, repeating this dose every five to seven days. When the season begins, hyposensitization already attained to the increasing pollen in the air may not be sufficient to prevent symptoms, and a reduction in dosage to 0.10 to 0.40 cc. of the 1 to 50 dilution every few days or to smaller doses, as described under co-seasonal therapy may be necessary. Treatment may also be stopped, to be resumed the following year.

2. *Perennial therapy* is favored by many allergists. With it treatment may be started at any time of year with small doses as described below if started during the season. After maximum doses have been reached, they may be repeated at seven- to fourteen-day intervals throughout the year with more frequent and possibly smaller doses during the pollination seasons according to the relief obtained. With such continued therapy for two or more years, hyposensitization is usually more permanent, skin reactions to the pollens may diminish or nearly disappear and the patient may finally be able to tolerate the maximum doses even during pollen seasons. Such perennial therapy offers more likelihood of eventual freedom from clinical symptoms without continued hyposensitization therapy than when pre-seasonal treatment alone is given. With such therapy, however, the pollen antigen may have to be changed from time to time since new pollen allergies may arise, either to pollens formerly unproductive of allergy, or to new pollens encountered in areas more frequently visited. As in all allergic therapy, absolute and prolonged coöperation of the patient with his intelligent understanding of the problem confronted by the physician is imperative.

3. *Co-seasonal therapy* is necessary for the control of symptoms arising during the pollen season. With small doses of the antigen, varying from 0.10 cc. of a 1 to 500 to 0.10 cc. of a 1 to 500,000 or more dilute according to the number of pollens in the antigen and the patient's degree of sensitization, given every day for five to ten days, symptoms are often controlled, providing the specific pollens to which the patient is exposed are included. As symptoms disappear, the doses can be increased by the physician and given less frequently according to the results.

The *length of pollen therapy*, as already stated, depends on the degree of sensitization, the number of pollens to which allergy exists, and the persistence of the hyposensitization which therapy creates. Each patient is a rule unto himself. Unfortunately, some patients must receive a varying amount of treatment for several years and some may need protection for an indefinite period in the same way that diabetics require insulin therapy throughout life.

Self-administration of Pollen Antigens.—This is justifiable under the following conditions: If small daily doses are indicated during co-seasonal treatment, and if the physician has determined that the dose does not produce undesirable local or general reactions, the patient may administer such an amount himself. Perennial therapy at regular intervals with the same amount of antigen, which dose has been found to produce no unfavorable reactions in the patient, may also be given by the patient if the physician so advises. If the patient's work prevents regular and necessary visits to the office, and especially if he lives miles away from the nearest physician, the patient may also administer the antigens. *He should report to the physician at regular intervals either by mail or in person and should only be given one dilution of the antigen at a time to decrease the possibility of a general reaction. Whenever self-administration of any antigen is allowed, the physician must instruct the patient or other person* who is to give the injections so that the syringe is correctly sterilized, the antigen accurately measured in a good tuberculin syringe, the skin cleaned and disinfected properly, and the injection given subcutaneously in an area free from underlying large veins. The patient must be provided with a schedule of doses so that a proper increase can be made, providing local reactions are not larger than 2 inches in diameter within twelve hours after injection, and providing general reactions, as described below, or exaggeration or reactivation of symptoms does not occur. When the patient is giving his solutions, the dilutions should be so weak and the speed of increase so slow that constitutional reactions are practically impossible. The control of general reactions is described below. *Self-administration of antigens, therefore, is only justifiable under the above circumstances and when the physician has given the above instructions.*

General Reactions and Their Control.—While pollen therapy is being given by the physician and when it, at times, needs to be self-administered, *it is most necessary for the patient to recognize indications of too large doses of antigen and the symptoms of the so-called general reaction.* Increased congestion and watering of the eyes and nose, sneezing, coughing, tightness and wheezing in the chest and actual asthma may develop within a few minutes to one hour after the injection according to the degree of the patient's pollen allergy. Cutaneous symptoms may also arise, including puffiness of the eyes and face, redness, itching and actual hives and swellings of varying areas of the body. With severe reactions, abdominal cramping and pain, and even bladder spasm and involuntary urination may occur. These reactions are more common during the pollen season for which reason doses of antigens must be increased very cautiously and frequently reduced as described above in co-seasonal therapy. When pollen therapy is carefully regulated, the likelihood of general reactions is greatly diminished. They are more apt to occur during the first year of treatment, especially in very sensitive patients. After an injection, the patient must wait in the physician's office for a few minutes up to fifteen to thirty minutes according to his susceptibility. *If any indications of a general reaction noted above arise, the physician must give from 0.1 to 0.8 cc. of 1 to 1000 epinephrine solution subcutaneously according to the degree of reaction and the age of the patient, and this dose must be repeated every five to sixty minutes until relief occurs and persists.* With severe reactions, such epinephrine may be necessary several times during the next twenty-four hours. If the reaction is severe, the placing of a tourniquet above the site of the injection, releasing it for one minute every four to five minutes over a period of twenty to thirty minutes retards the speed of antigen absorption and the degree of the general reaction. During pollen therapy, the patient may well carry 6 capsules containing $\frac{3}{8}$ grain of ephedrine in his pocket. If a reaction develops after leaving the physician's office, he should take 1 or 2 by mouth and immediately return to the office for the epinephrine therapy.

When self-administration of pollen antigens is indicated, the patient must be instructed about possible general reactions and must be provided with ampules of 1 to 1000 epinephrine and be instructed about the proper dose and its administration to counteract such symptoms. For one-half hour or so after an injection of antigen, the patient should remain at home and be able to give such epinephrine hypodermically if a general reaction develops.

Such reactions are much less common than several years ago since treatment is now started with small doses which fail to cause any exaggeration of symptoms, the doses are increased more carefully and doses are reduced, especially during the pollen season if any undue local or general reactivity arises. *At no time, it must again be emphasized, should pollen therapy exaggerate or reproduce the patient's symptoms.*

ANIMAL EMANATIONS

The dander from animals consisting of the cutaneous scales and the small amount of dust and particles from the hair may produce allergy in man. *Patients become sensitive to those emanations to which they are most frequently exposed, either from the live animals or from hair in carpets, rugs, upholstery, and bedding in the home, places of recreation or in automobiles.* Information concerning all such contacts, therefore, is most important in the patient's environmental history. Allergy to the emanations of horses, cows, cattle, cats, and dogs is most common because of their predominance on the farms or in the living environments. Cats and dogs in adjoining yards may give off emanations which blow into the home. The emanations of animals brought into the home on the clothes of the patient's relatives or friends are a definite source of trouble. The use of horse hair in mattresses and upholstery, the use of cattle and cow hair in pads under carpets and in some upholstery must be remembered. Patients become so sensitive to the emanations of horses, cats, and dogs that symptoms arise even on entering a house where their emanations are. The presence of cats or dogs in the basement or in a distant room may result in enough of their allergens in other parts of the house to affect the very sensitive patient. *Their former presence in houses years before may have left traces of emanations which cause such difficulty. Horses, far distant* from a house or in a field past which the sensitive patient rides in an automobile may cause allergic symptoms. *Wool allergy* is most severe in those who raise and handle sheep or who sell or prepare the crude wool for the markets or for the manufacture of yarn. It also occurs to the dusts of woolen blankets, fabrics, and especially of carpets, demanding environmental elimination and often hyposensitization therapy. *Goat hair* in mohair fabrics, *camel* and other hairs in garments and floor coverings give rise to allergy. Those working with *wild animals in zoos and circuses* develop sensitizations to their emanations. Hunters sensitized to *deer or other game dander* may be affected as they carry or handle the actual game or ride in automobiles or are in homes where the skins or stuffed heads or animals have been. Allergy to *rodents such as mice, rats, marmots* in or under the house or to *squirrels, rabbits,* and similar animals develop according to the frequency and degree of exposure. Laboratory workers who inhale the emanations of mice, guinea pigs, rabbits, monkeys, dogs, or cats may become sensitized. Sensitization to the furs of various animals sold commercially occurs. Inhalant sensitizations to the

dusts given off by them, however, are not as common as are
contact reactions on the skin. Such dermatitis is most frequently
due to the dyes and chemicals used in the curing and manufacturing of the furs, since the processing of them eliminates nearly all
the dusts naturally arising from them.

Allergy to the dust and emanations from birds is common. Raisers
of poultry and birds of all types may develop sensitivity to specific
ones. Sensitization to canaries or parrots or to the dust from
stuffed birds develops with varying frequency. The emanations
from canaries especially may blow through the house from the
room in which the birds are or from an aviary in the yard. Emanations from birds roosting or nesting in vines or trees near bedroom
windows or on roofs or eaves of the house may cause allergy.
Sensitization to feathers is frequent because of their use in pillows,
upholstery, comforters, and mattresses. When present, the removal of all sources of them from the patient's environment is
most important. Or the pillows and mattresses used by the
patient may be covered with allergen-proof slips or covers. Patients who have slept on feather or down mattresses especially may
be allergic thereto. The removal of such mattresses from the
house and the thorough cleaning of the living environments as
discussed on page 31, of course, is most necessary.

SILK

*Silk sensitization arises at all ages and is often associated with a
high degree of allergy as evidenced by a large scratch reaction.* The
frequency of inhalant allergy in those raising silk worms and in
those gathering cocoons and in spinners of silk fiber therefrom is
not known. Dermatitis in silk handlers, however, has been described for several centuries. The very allergic individual may
develop severe nasobronchial symptoms or dermatitis from the
inhalation of the traces of silk allergen in the air of a room in
which silk curtains or other silk fabrics are, or in which women
who are wearing silk have been, or are at present. Silk underwear
or bedclothes or silk in the dust of rooms must be suspected in
such patients. One girl with a generalized dermatitis all over the
body, even in the scalp, associated with severe pruritus, was gradually relieved when all silk furnishings or clothing, including stockings, were removed from herself and her mother and hyposensitization therapy, starting with minute doses of a silk antigen, was
given. The processing and the dyeing of the silk cloth and fabric
probably modify the silk allergens to a certain degree.

ORRIS ROOT, KARAYA GUM AND OTHER INGREDIENTS OF COSMETICS

Orris root powder made from dried iris bulbs is light in weight, has a delicate odor, and is used in certain face powders. It is also used to dry shampoo the hair. Varying degrees of nasal and bronchial allergy arises from its inhalation and a hive-like dermatitis may develop when used in a face powder. Severe symptoms may arise causing profuse coryza, sneezing, nasal blocking, ocular congestion, or severe allergic bronchitis or bronchial asthma with the slightest exposure. One patient was unable to go into theaters or homes where orris containing powders were in use until hyposensitization was accomplished. Sensitizations to new ingredients may arise as shown by the hairdresser who first developed nasal allergy to orris root and later to rye and rice flours used to dry shampoo the hair. *Rice powder, dyes, various perfumes, and rarely other ingredients in powders and cosmetics* give rise to nasobronchial and cutaneous allergic manifestations. *Contact allergy to the dyes* and other ingredients in lip sticks cause eruptions on the lips known as *cheilitis.* Patch tests on the skin in susceptible individuals with various preparations will reveal the ones to which allergy exists. Rouges, mascara, and various eyelash and eyebrow dyes may also produce eruptions, at times producing conjunctival inflammation and even corneal ulceration.

Various ingredients in *hair setting solutions* not only cause eruptions in the scalp and the skin of the neck and face, and on the hands of the operator, but also nasal and bronchial allergy in the patron and the operator herself. The dried *karaya gum* (see page 98) in the hair used so frequently in such solutions is prone to develop such sensitizations. *Acacia (gum arabic), gum tragacanth, linseed gum and quince seed gum* used in such preparations may also give rise to allergy. One case of asthma from the inhalation of acacia dust from a factory was reported. One operator who had severe sneezing and watering of the nose from the dried karaya gum in the hair and in the air of her salon was successfully hyposensitized.

PYRETHRUM AND DERRIS ROOT

Pyrethrum is composed of powdered leaves of a daisy closely related to the chrysanthemum. It is commonly used as an insect powder or insecticide and gives rise to nasobronchial and cutaneous allergies of varying severities. Carpets and rugs during manufacture and also when demothed are frequently thoroughly sprayed with it, and furniture and theater seats in public places often receive such an application.   One recorded patient developed a severe and fatal attack of asthma from the inhalation of pyrethrum in the air of a theater.   Most commercial fly sprays contain pyrethrum.

Allergy to *derris root* used in insecticides has recently been described indicating the advisability of its use in skin testing.

GLUE

The inhalation of glue dust may produce nasobronchial and cutaneous allergy which at times is of an extreme severity.   Skin reactions by the scratch test may be large; intradermal tests should never be done before scratch tests are tried.   Such patients are so sensitive that the glue dust in the air of offices, libraries, and the homes where books and furniture are which have had glue used in their manufacture will cause difficulty.   One patient with generalized eczema all over the body preventing sleep for months and incapacitating him for two years was glue sensitive and was gradually relieved with hyposensitization, at first with infinitesimal doses.   Glue made from fish is most frequently productive of allergy.   Glue sensitive patients are usually sensitive to and give large reactions to various fish allergens.   However, glue of animal origin is also causative of allergic reactivity.   Labels covered with glue may cause symptoms when sensitized patients lick them. Postage stamps, however, rarely are treated with such glues. Glue sensitive patients may develop local and general reactions from the allergen absorbed from the glue on the inner soles of shoes.   Further discussion of glue allergy is on page 76.

COTTONSEED AND KAPOK

Cottonseed allergen produces severe sensitization in certain patients so that the dust from cotton linters used in mattresses, pillows, upholstery, and even the minute amount of the allergen in cotton fabrics will cause nasobronchial, ocular, and cutaneous manifestations.   Cottonseed meal in fowl, cattle, and cow feeds is especially dangerous when inhaled by the individual sensitized to this allergen.   Cottonseed allergy must be remembered in workers in cotton fields, in those engaged in cottonseed oil mills and in others who contact this product in the industries.   Allergy to the liquid and hydrogenated oils will be discussed under Ingestants.

Kapok allergen in the dust of the seeds of the floss, itself, also causes similar allergic manifestations.   Those patients sensitized

to cottonseed or to kapok may or may not be allergic to the other
allergen. Allergens common to both and specific for each one
explain such individual or common reactivity. The silk floss
which comes from the large pods of the kapok trees so commonly
used in pillows, mattresses and upholstery, contain varying
amounts of the sensitizing allergens. Such floss pulverizes with
age and often sensitizes patients who are exposed. That there
is probably as much kapok and cottonseed allergy as feather
allergy, has become apparent in recent years. The use of allergen-
proof covers or other non-allergenic materials for sensitized patients was discussed on page 327. The gradual development of
new allergens in ageing old kapok and cotton linters will be discussed below.

HOUSE DUSTS

House dust sensitizations have been stressed for twenty years as
causes of nasobronchial, ocular, and cutaneous allergies. Certain
investigators have held that an unknown allergen in such dust is
responsible for much of the allergy arising therefrom. The recent
discovery by Cohen of such an allergen in old kapok or cotton
linters aged in tight jars which, with the contained fibers, had been
autoclaved at a high temperature, lends credence to this idea.
However, house dusts also contain many allergens from carpets,
pads, upholstery, glue, wall paper, clothes, cosmetics, animals,
pollens, air-borne, and from flowers and blooms in the house and
in the air coming through the windows and doors, insecticides,
and many other obvious sources. Such ingredients, of course,
vary with each home. The dusts of hotels, theaters, and public
places also give rise to allergy and their varying content of allergens
is obvious. Inhalant sensitive patients usually give reactions to
one or more stock house dust extracts by the scratch and, especially, by the intradermal tests. When such are present, particularly, if reactions to animal emanations, kapok, cottonseed, orris
root, pyrethrum, silk, or other miscellaneous allergens or to pollens are at all marked, the control of such specific allergies will
often make hyposensitization with dust extracts unnecessary.
Environmental control as described on page 31, however, is most
important in such patients.

When house dust hyposensitization is indicated, the *treatment*
with autogenous dust extracts from the patient's living environments
is more desirable than with stock dust extracts. The dust may be
taken from the bag of a vacuum cleaner after the cleaning of all
the carpets, overstuffed furniture and mattresses, or separate

specimens of dust from single rooms, special carpets, pieces of furniture or mattresses may be obtained. After extracts are made, skin testing usually indicates the degree of allergy, and treatment with single or combined extracts can be given. A marked reaction to the dust of one room or carpet or piece of furniture may lead to the discovery of the major or of one important source of inhalant allergy. However, small or negative reactions may be associated with definite clinical allergy.

OCCUPATIONAL AND RECREATIONAL DUSTS

Sensitization to the allergens in the dusts of any environment frequented by the patient, of course, is possible. Again nasobronchial, ocular, and cutaneous manifestations are common results though occasional gastro-intestinal allergy, allergic toxemia, and migraine or other central nervous system allergy may arise as described on page 132. *Every office, professional, mercantile, industrial, or out-of-door occupation obviously exposes the individual to various air-borne and contact allergens which need recognition* and study in the patient whose problem is difficult to understand and control. Likewise, *recreations*, be they golf, tennis, hunting, hiking, gardening, botanizing, wood working, photography, or any other, offer specific challenges from the allergic viewpoint. Tests with specially obtained or prepared inhalant allergens or substances productive of possible contact sensitization, must be carried out by the physician.

HAY, GRAIN, AND FEED DUSTS

Individuals who are around barns or farms where animals or fowl are fed may become sensitized to the dusts of hay, grain, and other feeds. This is especially true of patients who are prone to develop inhalant allergies to pollens or animal emanations. The type of hay, of course, varies in every area. Timothy, red top, orchard grass, and clover, are cultivated commonly where winters are cold; oats and barley in the warmer regions, and any of many other grasses are contained in the hay of other areas. Alfalfa, especially where irrigation is available, is common and gives rise to allergy. Hay dust, itself, contains allergens other than pollens to which allergy develops. The resins of grasses and of weeds, as discussed on page 121, may give rise to contact allergy. The spores of fungi, smuts, and molds or small amounts of animal emanations or insect pests in the hay may cause reactions in sensitized patients. Therefore, extracts of various hays are advisable

4

for routine testing of patients exposed to hay, and extracts of various hays from the patient's own barn or stacks may be useful for his study.

Allergy *to wheat, barley, oats, rye, corn, rice, or other grain products, to various bean products, cottonseed meal, flaxseed, or other foods must be suspected in certain patients.* Stock or specially prepared extracts of such are important for testing the patient. The mixed and *prepared feeds for cows, cattle, and fowl, particularly the chicken mashes,* have varying contents which must be known to the patient's physician. The frequency of cottonseed and flaxseed in them is important to keep in mind. Chicken raisers are subject to allergy from the dusts of feeds which may contain corn, wheat, barley, alfalfa, sardine meal, coconut, bone meal, yeast, cod-liver oil, molasses, and other similar ingredients. Such airborne allergens may blow for several miles and cause symptoms in patients distant from the chicken farms themselves.

FLOURS AND DUSTS FROM OTHER FOODS

Bakers, especially, but also cooks, grocers, and those working in flour mills may become sensitive to inhaled flours of varying types. Since wheat flour is most commonly handled in this country, it most frequently produces allergy. Other flours are also inhaled by mill workers, which may account for sensitizations which are usually found to other cereal grains, though group allergens in the closely related grains are a possible reason. In sensitized patients, large skin reactions by the scratch test are usually obtained, though, as in all types of allergy, skin tests may be negative. It is surprising that more bakers who inhale such large amounts of these cereal dusts for years, do not become sensitized. Their constant exposure without fairly long vacations may account for this. Even though vacations occur, some flour dust must remain in the bronchial tract for days or probably weeks. Most sensitized people, especially bakers, must be carefully protected with masks and with prolonged desensitization if tolerance is to be obtained. Some are impossible to hyposensitize. One baker with bronchial asthma and large skin reactions to wheat and other cereal grains was relieved by a cereal-free diet so that he could inhale the flours with no difficulty.

Handlers of other foods may become sensitized to the inhalation of allergens therefrom. Allergy to spices, especially pepper, to fish, vegetables, and fruits have occasionally arisen through inhalation of mere traces in the air. One nurse developed hay fever when she entered a home where grapefruit were on the dining room table. Another patient rapidly had hives when at a table on which there was cauliflower or cabbage. The vapor and odor of certain vegetables and especially of fish and eggs, have been known to produce allergic manifestations.

DRUGS AND MEDICAMENTS

Patients may be so allergic to *various drugs* that their inhalation in minute amounts gives rise to allergic manifestations. Such portal of entry is not so common for drugs as is the gastrointestinal tract or the skin. Druggists especially, through inhalation, may develop symptoms from ipecac. The inhalation of salvarsan has resulted in dermatitis. Other drugs through inhalation occasionally may result in allergic symptomatology.

FLY AND INSECT EMANATIONS

Allergy to the emanations of lake flies, as reported to the "May Fly" by Figley and to the "Caddis Fly" by Parlato, may produce serious nasal and bronchial symptoms. The writer has observed similar cases at Clear Lake in California. Likewise, emanations of butterflies, moths, gnats, and other flies are so abundant in the air in certain areas in hot weather that allergic symptoms develop. Hyposensitization with specific extracts gives good results. Other types of allergy to insect allergens, especially from bites and stings, will be described later.

SPORES OF FUNGI AND SMUTS

Allergy to the *spores of fungi* which are their germinal elements and about one-twentieth the size of pollens causes nasobronchial, cutaneous and probably other tissue reactions. Over 5000 species of fungi, including molds and yeasts have been identified. They are distributed everywhere, present even to a depth of 4 feet below the surface of the earth and abundant in the air even, in small numbers, at 7000 feet. In the ground, they break down organic substances, especially cellulose and wood and, assimilating various nitrogenous and mineral compounds, they fix them in the soil. Surrounding certain roots, organic matter is broken down and made available for the plant. The outside air contains from 100 to 4000 or more spores of fungi per cc. and extremely high counts may be in the air in certain rooms. *Cheeses* are made with the aid of special molds, species of penicilium being responsible for Camembert and Roquefort. *Yeasts*, of course, are necessary in the manufacture of breads, beer, and wine.

Much experience is necessary for the *accurate classification of fungi*. An idea of the number of species of spores present in the air can be obtained by exposing sterile media in Petri dishes for brief periods to the air. Tightly covered after exposure, the spores gradually grow at room temperatures on such media and in a few days or longer, the visible and microscopic appearances allow classification. Plants, trees, and vegetables are prone to have specific fungi. Moreover, the degree of moisture, the climate, the nature of the soil, and particularly the type of vegetation in an area determine the kind of spores present in the air. As a result of spore counts by various students in America, the most frequent spores are known. Patients suspected of fungus allergy are usually tested routinely with 15 to 20 such allergens. *Smuts which grow in grains may also produce allergy* and routine testing with the important ones is desirable. Media may also be exposed in areas around or inside the patient's home and autogenous fungus extracts can be prepared for testing and therapy. Some of the most common fungi, according to Fineburg, are alternaria, hormodendrum (cladosporium), helminthosporium, aspergillus, penicillium, mucor, rhizopus, saccharomyces (yeast), chætomium, monilia, trichoderma, fusarium, smut, and trichophyton.

Yeasts are fungi which maintain a unicellular growth and have no mycelia. Routine testing of all patients with yeasts is important. Patients not only inhale yeasts but ingest relatively large amounts in bread, raised bakery products, including white crackers, graham crackers, rye crisp, and especially in beer. Yeast is further discussed on page 93.

TOBACCO ALLERGY

Many people become aware of their intolerance to tobacco, and it is probable that most of these idiosyncratic reactions are allergic in nature. *Sensitization to allergens in the tobacco or possibly in the paper or other ingredients of cigarettes or in various essential oils, perfumes, and flavors added to pipe or chewing tobacco, causes, reactivity in various tissues of the body. It may well be that the main damage of tobacco, therefore, resides in allergy, rather than in toxic effects of nicotine or of the various combustion products.* Many investigations, especially by Harkavy and Sulzberger, have been made on skin reactions to tobacco allergens. Patients may react to one kind of tobacco and not to another. Skin reactions are obtained in a large number of individuals, including children who have been exposed to tobacco smoke. Tobacco allergy, in common with other inhalant and ingestant allergies, probably primarily affects the vascular tissues. It may be that the contraction of the capillaries in the fingernail bed which can be seen with a capillary microscope after the inhalation of tobacco smoke in many persons, is due to allergic reactivity. It is generally agreed that the serious affection of the extremities, called endarteritis obliterans, is due to arterial allergy, usually to tobacco. Eczema and other dermatoses, especially of the face, neck, and hands, may arise from tobacco allergy. Allergy of the blood-vessels may be responsible for some increase in high blood-pressure, headache, dizziness, and other symptoms not definitely associated with tobacco allergy today. Various gastro-intestinal symptoms, including peptic ulcer, may arise or be increased by this type of sensitization. Good results with desensitization to tobacco allergens apparently arise in certain patients.

CHEMICAL INHALANTS

Allergy occasionally develops to *air-borne chlorine, phenol, lysol, ether, chloroform, formaldehyde, and other chemical substances*. Even the brief smell of them may cause allergic symptoms. Acting as haptens, as explained on page 26, these chemicals unite with body proteins and cause specific sensitization. A nurse developed allergic dermatitis from air-borne chlorine twenty years ago and gradually sensitizations to all the other chemical "odors" so that work was impossible in hospital, office, or home when the odors of any of these chemicals could be detected by the patient. Attempted hyposensitization, first with infinitesimal amounts, has failed to increase tolerance. *Naphthalene, used in moth balls and as an insecticide in gardens* has produced asthma and dermatitis in two patients. Allergy developing from the ingestion, skin contact and therapeutic injection of various chemicals and drugs will be discussed later. The fact that allergic reactions may arise from such chemicals, even in the minutest amounts, giving rise to mild, hardly discernible symptoms or more definite or serious manifestations, shows the great unknown possibilities of allergic reactivities to substances of all types.

INGESTANTS

FOOD ALLERGY

Foods probably produce more allergic manifestations in various tissues of the body than does any other group of allergens. This is due, in part, to the continuous daily ingestion of foods, often in excessive amounts. Local or contact allergy may arise from foods in the mucous membrane of the gastro-intestinal tract similar to the poison oak type of reaction, as discussed on page 127. Most of the symptoms, however, occur in the sensitized nasobronchial, ocular, cutaneous, nervous, vascular, gastro-intestinal, urological, or other tissues from the blood-borne food allergens absorbed through the gastro-intestinal mucosa. As formerly explained, all tissue cells of the body are sensitized more or less, the symptoms depending on the tissues or organs which have the greatest degree of sensitization.

Symptoms From Causes Other Than Allergy.—*Gastro-intestinal symptoms, headaches, and other less definite disturbances may arise from many other causes than allergy.* The fact that gastro-intestinal symptoms occur in appendicitis, gall-bladder disease, peptic ulcer, cancer, rectal disease, chronic diseases such as nephritis, diabetes, anemia, and many other diseased states must be kept in mind. The patient often connects such symptoms with the eating or imagined effect of some food. Without a careful examination and laboratory studies by the physician, the symptoms may incorrectly be attributed to food allergy. *Foods eaten in excess or when fatigued or nervous* may also produce gastro-intestinal symptoms which must not be attributed to allergy. *Unwarranted aversions for foods* due to whims or fancies or to familial habits of eating explains certain dislikes or apparent disagreements in certain patients. *All this emphasizes again the necessity of a thorough study of the patient for all possible causes of symptoms before food allergy is considered to be the only likely etiology.*

Frequency.—*Everyone is susceptible to food as well as to some other type of allergy in varying degrees.* Analysis of the histories of large groups of the population, especially by Vaughan, have shown that 60 per cent gave past or present histories of allergy, that probable food sensitization was evident in 62 per cent, inhalant allergy in 23 per cent, and contact sensitization in 14 per cent. Such histories do not elicit all evidences of allergy throughout life. Thus even a larger number of people is undoubtedly susceptible to food, as well as to inhalant and contact allergens. Moreover, when it is remembered that most infections produce rashes and other symptoms due to allergy, it is obvious that few, if any, people die without developing various types and numbers of allergic reactivities. *This general tendency to allergy,* however, *is exaggerated and increased when allergy is present in the relatives of one side,* and *especially if present in both sides of the family. Moreover, there is a definite inherited tendency for a manifestation of allergy such as bronchial asthma, eczema, or migraine or recurrent* *headaches to run through families.*   Also, the tendency to develop food, pollen, or even animal emanation sensitizations is transmitted in certain families and at times the tendency to develop allergy to specific foods may recur in close relatives.   Thus, egg, milk, wheat, fish, or nut allergy may be found in several generations.

Why Allergy Develops.—No additional information is available to answer the question, *"Why does allergy develop?"*   Predisposition through inheritance and excessive or intermittent exposures, inhalations, or ingestions of the allergenic substance are the most potent influences.   Deficiencies in vitamin intake, especially of vitamin C have been suspected, but proof that this and that other glandular or chronic diseased states influence the onset of allergy is lacking.

Food and other types of allergy may occur at any time of life. When the family history, particularly of food allergy, is marked, food sensitivity may appear soon after birth and gastro-intestinal symptoms and later eczema may be real problems, as discussed on page 119.   As age increases, hyposensitization or tolerance to the allergenic foods often increases and manifestations such as eczema, gastro-intestinal allergy, or bronchial asthma may disappear.   Such relief is not always persistent, however, and usually the manifestations continue or the food allergy remains potentially active, ready to cause the same or other symptoms at a later age. Food sensitizations may develop in late childhood, in adolescence, or adult life.   The writer has studied several patients who, in their fifties, sixties, or even later, have for the first time developed bronchial asthma or eczema from food sensitizations.

Food allergy may originally arise to one food such as egg or milk. Gradually, however, other sensitizations usually develop, according to the degree of inherited propensity.   In a few patients, large numbers of foods are productive of allergy and in a rare patient, allergy apparently is present to practically all foods in varying degrees of intensity.

In addition to the inherited propensity to develop allergy, especially to foods, the *eating of large amounts of a given food day after day or at separated intervals, tends toward sensitization thereto.* Eating of certain foods during digestive upsets or when fatigued or taking them with practically no other food, may tend toward allergy.   Thus in infancy, especially with a family history of allergy particularly to foods, it is well to gradually increase new foods in the diet and to continue the feeding of any new foods every day or two for long periods.   If such foods are stopped for two or more weeks, infants may become sensitized as are experimental animals two or more weeks after a single preparatory injection or the feeding of food or other allergens. Allergy to foods possibly may be delayed or modified in susceptible infants when there is a marked familial history of allergy in one or both parents and relatives, if before or during conception the father's and mother's allergies are adequately controlled through diet and other therapeutic measures and if during pregnancy the mother's allergies are properly treated. The infant, after birth, moreover, must have its allergies controlled and, if food allergy is active in the progenitors, eggs, wheat, and possibly milk, should be replaced by other foods, during the first six to twelve months. Longer exclusion of eggs may be advisable.

Degree, Time of Onset, and Duration of Reaction.—*The symptoms arising from the ingestion of an allergenic food may occur in a few minutes or in one to three days after its ingestion.* When a marked allergy is present, the symptoms may be immediate, at times extremely severe, even being associated with weakness, exhaustion, and collapse. Immediate symptoms occur when the reacting bodies are widely distributed through the body tissues and scratch reactions, as discussed on page 23, are easily obtained. When less severe allergy is present, the symptoms are usually delayed one or more hours in their onset. *At times, the eating of the food two or more days in succession is necessary to break down temporary tolerance and produce symptoms.* In these patients skin tests may be negative or indefinite. The severity of the symptoms depends on the degree of the patient's allergy and the amount of the food ingested. The mere trace or even the smell of a food in very allergic patients may produce severe symptoms. This necessitates the entire exclusion of any such food from the diet and great care with which meals must be cooked, as discussed in Chapter V. When symptoms arise, they are due to food allergens brought by the blood to the sensitized cells, be they in the lungs, skin, brain or other parts of the body. *It is probable that such allergens remain in these cells at times for long periods, possibly in some patients for several weeks or longer.* More-over, an ingested food remains in decreasing amounts in the intestinal tract for one to two weeks. All the while, food allergens are being absorbed to a decreasing degree and are probably attracted and held by cells in the body tissues, especially where the major sensitization exists. All of these possible factors and conditions influence the degree and the duration of allergic symptoms.

Cyclic Recurrences.—*Symptoms arising from food allergy and to a lesser extent from inhalant allergens, tend to recur in cyclic explo-*

sive attacks. This is due to the so-called refractoriness or desensitization which develops after symptoms have existed for a few hours to several days. During the attack, the reacting bodies which have increasingly bound themselves to the cells of those tissues where the major allergic reactivity resides are exhausted and disappear. Then for days or weeks thereafter, the causative allergen may be eaten or inhaled without symptoms. Gradually the reacting bodies, comparable to the antibodies of infection, again accumulate in the shock tissues and then, with gradual or possibly sudden onset, the symptoms may reoccur. Thus, the patient may eat the allergenic food or, less often, inhale the causative allergen continuously and only have his allergic manifestations such as bronchial asthma, nasal allergy, urticaria, recurrent headache or migraine once every month or two. *The patient may be potentially susceptible at other times, attacks being precipitated by secondary causes such as wind, cold, excitement, infections, and especially by menstruation in women.* These causes are further discussed on page 107. The termination of the attacks of bronchial asthma, especially in children, and also of recurrent headaches may be due to the abstinence from all food due to vomiting or refusal to eat, which often occurs. Gradually, as foods are again eaten, the attack recurs, according to the degree of sensitization which is present. This cyclic recurrent character of allergic manifestations is so important that a history of cyclic symptoms should always suggest allergy as an important etiological consideration.

Shock Organs.—*Patients may have allergic reactions in one organ or area of the body from one or more foods and reactions in other areas from other foods.* Thus one patient may have recurrent headaches due to allergy to wheat and onions, nasal allergy and particularly nasal congestion necessitating clearing the throat from milk, right-sided abdominal pain and soreness from oranges, lettuce and bananas, constipation and pruritus ani from wheat, apples and lemon. Then, again, one or usually a few foods in varying degrees may produce several different allergic manifestations.

Association With Inhalant and Infectant Allergies.—*The concomitance of food allergy with inhalant and, at times, infectant allergies, must always be remembered.* Some patients are affected with food allergy alone. However, the tendency to multiple types of sensitizations is the rule and most patients are best tested with all important food and inhalant allergens and their histories must be carefully analyzed from the viewpoint of all kinds of allergy. *Successful treatment usually necessitates the control of all important* *allergies.* Certain patients with minor food sensitizations are relieved thereof by the proper treatment of their inhalant allergies. Other patients with hay fever due to pollens are relieved by the elimination of allergenic foods.

Seasonal and Geographic Influences.—*Food allergy is definitely influenced by seasons and geographic locations.* Such influences on inhalant sensitizations have been discussed on page 38. *For many years, the writer has observed the beneficial effect that the summer months exert on many food allergies.* This benefit increases from mid April until the longest day and gradually decreases until the middle of August or September—approximately from one equinox to another. Tolerance for foods increases in many patients so that they can be taken without allergic reactions. Steadily, from August until December or January, tolerance for allergenic foods decreases, thereafter increasing again until June. The seasons do not so affect all food allergies, especially when they are marked in degree. The explanation of the favorable effect of the summer months probably resides in the increased amount of electrical and radiant energy available. Humidity, atmospheric pressure or ionization of air has failed to explain the benefit.

Food allergy also is diminished or inactivated in certain patients by residence in a dry and especially an inland area. In the San Francisco Bay area, the writer has had an unusual opportunity to arrive at this decision. Foods which cannot be tolerated without asthma, nasal blocking or eczema can be eaten with no symptoms 15 to 20 miles inland even on the river delta or in Contra Costa, Sonoma, Napa, or Lake Counties. When such patients, however, have their allergenic foods removed from their diets, they can remain on the ocean shore or near the bay without difficulty. Again, the true explanation of this effect is lacking. Altitude certainly is not responsible since benefit occurs in low areas such as Death Valley. So-called marine asthma has been described in Europe. The frequency of asthma along the ocean, especially in large cosmopolitan areas, has long been known. On the contrary, the benefit of desert climates and of residence in the dry inland plateau and the southwest of our country has attracted thousands of patients with nasal, bronchial and other chronic symptoms, many undoubtedly due in whole or in part to food sensitizations.

Food Dislikes and Disagreements.—Food dislikes and disagreements as reported by the patient must be noted by the physician since they may be indicative of food allergy. Many infants refuse to eat foods to which allergy exists and when eaten, vomiting, regurgitation, diarrhea, or other symptoms may arise. Many adults have an inherent distaste for allergenic foods and give a history of never having eaten milk, eggs, fish or other foods. It must be emphasized that *all such histories are not indicative of food allergies.* As stressed by Alvarez, Vaughan and others, these dislikes and disagreements are also due to fads or fancies established through habits of eating or other psychic influences. Gastro-intestinal or other constitutional disease may also be responsible, though the possibility of gastro-intestinal allergy must be remembered. Many patients, moreover, like foods and have had no self-recognized disturbances from foods which are found by the physician to be productive of definite allergy. *Thus, this history of food dislikes or disagreements is valuable from the diagnostic viewpoint, providing it is interpreted correctly by the trained physician.*

The diagnosis of food allergy has been discussed on page 21. In brief, the history, especially of possible food dislikes or idiosyncrasies, the interpretation of skin reactions to food allergens which are obtained and the important use of trial diet, have been discussed. The elimination diets for trial diagnostic study of such patients are described in Chapter V.

DESENSITIZATION

Food allergies tend to diminish in childhood, especially if the causative foods are eliminated from the diets. When mild allergies are present at any time of life, a few weeks or months may suffice to restore tolerance for weeks, months, or, at times, for years to come. In many patients, however, continued and complete elimination of such foods is necessary for one or several years and in others desensitization never occurs, or only partial tolerance is regained. Such tolerance for foods may last for weeks, months, or years, according to the ability of the tissues to hold the desensitization which has been established.

When allergies to important foods such as wheat, milk, or eggs, or to large numbers of important foods such as vegetables or fruits occur, *hypodermic administration of antigens* containing these allergenic foods has been tried by many physicians. *In general, such therapy has usually failed,* though some reports of success have been published. It may be that the administration of minute doses of antigen containing five to twelve allergens in dilutions of 1 to 50,000 or even weaker, given every day or so, being raised gradually according to the patient's response, may prove more beneficial. *Oral desensitization has also been successful in certain hands,* but generally this procedure has not been successful. *Thus, prolonged and accurate elimination of the causative foods for the present must be depended upon for possible desensitization and increased tolerance.*

DENATURIZATION OF FOODS

The allergens in foods are modified by varying degrees of heat and drying so that symptoms in the sensitized patient who ingests such foods are reduced or entirely prevented. For instance, many people develop hives or gastro-intestinal symptoms from uncooked but not from cooked fruits. Certain infants can take boiled and especially canned milk as reported by Ratner and not uncooked or pasteurized milk. Moreover, *modification of allergens seems to occur from the action of acids* as in lactic acid milk products. Such *tolerance for denaturized allergens*, however, *usually occurs in the mildly sensitive patient.* In the writer's practice, infants, children, and adults who are definitely sensitive to milk, wheat, or fruits usually necessitate total elimination of all such foods, even when they have been superheated for long periods. Thus the elimination diets as detailed in this volume make no use of denatured foods. When symptoms have been relieved, it is often wise to first add canned milk or cooked fruits until evidences of lack of allergy or increased tolerance are obtained.

This inability to entirely destroy allergenic activity by superheating is demonstrated by the failure to prevent scratch reactions with autoclaved allergens which in the unheated state have given large reactions in certain allergic patients.

BIOLOGICAL RELATIONSHIP OF FOODS

Vaughan and, later, Ellis have published a list of important foods according to biological relationships. These are to be found on page 222. *When a patient is clinically sensitive to one food, associated with or without a skin reaction, he may also be allergic to closely related foods.* Thus some patients have a group sensitization to all cereal grains, all legumes or to all citrus fruits. However, *this is not the rule since wheat, orange, or apricot allergy without sensitization to their biologically related foods frequently occurs.* As stated on page 13, when skin reactions occur, clinical allergy is not necessarily present and can only be assured by the actual feeding of suspected foods to the symptom-free patient.

TREATMENT OF FOOD ALLERGY

Increase in tolerance to the eliminated foods, by the natural tendency—especially in children—to become less sensitive, and, finally, by hypodermic or oral desensitization, has been discussed above.

When symptoms occur from food, as well as other types of allergy, *epinephrine is indicated.* It is given hypodermically in doses of 0.1 to 0.8 cc. of a 1 to 1000 dilution every five to thirty minutes according to severity and repeated every hour if necessary for relief. It is valuable, especially in bronchial asthma, urticaria, or angioneurotic edema, and may be tried when acute gastro-intestinal allergy or allergic migraine are suspected.

Epinephrine, 1 to 100, may be vaporized by a special glass atomizer and inhaled for relief of mild bronchial asthma and for mild pruritus and possibly for other mild allergic manifestations (see page 113). Actual droplets of this strong epinephrine must not enter the mouth and be swallowed since severe gastric pain and distress may occur. Thus, the mouth may be rinsed with water after such inhalations.

Attempts to change or reduce food sensitizations by *peptone therapy given by mouth or hypodermically have failed in practically all cases. The hastening of enhancement of gastric or intestinal digestion* by the use of dilute hydrochloric acid, pepsin, pancreatin, or bile salts *has yielded no definite results.* Non-specific therapy with injections of milk, vaccines, and also of blood drawn from the patient have been disappointing in the control of food allergy.

Recently *histamine,* given hypodermically or in small doses and slowly by vein, has controlled some manifestations of food allergy (see page 132). *Histaminase,* a ferment which breaks down histamine by mouth and hypodermically, has failed to decrease food allergy except in a few cases (see page 125).

FOODS AND CONDIMENTS*

Origin, Habitat, and Biological Relationship. — *Though allergy can develop to any food, it is most common to those foods eaten in large amounts nearly every day or intermittently with periods of two or more weeks intervening. Certain foods, moreover, tend to produce severe allergy.* This is true of egg, milk, wheat, fin and shell fish, buckwheat, celery, onion, peanuts, bananas, and cottonseed products. As already discussed on page 62, *foods of closely related species probably contain group allergens as well as specific allergens which cause sensitization.* Thus, a *patient may be allergic to several closely related foods with a predominant sensitization to one of them. Allergy to one food without any reactivity*

* For much of this information, I am indebted to Vaughan, W. C., The Practice of Allergy, St. Louis, C. V. Mosby Co., 1939.

to closely related foods occurs possibly more frequently than do such group reactions. This tendency to the development of group allergies also exists in all other types of allergy. For example, in pollen allergy sensitization to nearly all graminæ pollens of varying genuses and species is common. The classification of vegetable and animal foods, according to family, genus and species will be found on page 222. Some experimental study of these specific and group allergens has been made, though their existence depends nearly entirely on clinical evidence. *Further experimental investigation of these allergens in closely related foods is urgently needed. The effect of heat and drying on food allergens,* as discussed on page 60, *must be kept in mind as foods and menus are ordered and prepared for the food sensitive individual.*

CEREALS

Those carbohydrate foods obtained from the seeds of grasses are called cereal grains. They include wheat, rice, corn, barley, oats, and rye. As noted above, patients may be sensitive to one or more with or without sensitizations to the other related ones. The grain that is eaten most commonly produces most allergy. Thus, wheat is certainly the chief offender in America, whereas rice in Japan and rye in the Scandinavian countries are probably the chief causes of allergy.

Wheat (triticum sativum) has been favored for several thousand years for food since it is pleasant to the taste and is more easily leavened than any other cereal flour, due to its gliadin content. Over 300 varieties of wheat have been developed, varying in softness and hardness. Two kinds of flour, namely graham or whole wheat and patent or white flour, are in use. A physician, Sylvester Graham, about 1850 recommended the whole wheat flour to which his name was given.

Wheat is used in the making of practically all commercial breads, bakery products, pies, cookies, cakes, many dried and commercial breakfast foods, macaroni, spaghetti, vermicelli, noodles, gravies, sauces, thickened soups and creamed foods. Commercial rye and buckwheat flours and probably many soy, lima bean, rice, corn, and potato flours contain wheat. Unleavened bread or the Matzoth of the Jewish Passover is a wheat wafer with no yeast.

Patients, therefore, must know every ingredient of all prepared foods and also the composition of the flours and other products used, in order to be certain that all wheat, egg, milk, or other forbidden foods are excluded. The frequency of allergy to yeast

—at times to one species of yeast—is discussed on page 93. This, at times, requires the elimination of yeast raised bakery products and the use of baking powder for such foods. The presence of other yeast and fungi in bread and bakery products as in all other foods, as evidenced by the growth of such fungi therein with suitable moisture and warmth, may produce allergy in occasional individuals. Various foods containing wheat are listed on pages 231 to 233.

Rye (secale cereale) has been used for food probably as long as has wheat. It will grow in colder climates than will wheat, especially in northern Russia, Scandinavia, Germany, the Dakotas, Minnesota, and Wisconsin. It contains less gliadin and thus leavens less easily. Commercial rye flours usually contain wheat to diminish the heaviness and strong flavor of pure rye bread. Rye bread nearly always contains wheat. Even the dark pumpernickel bread may contain wheat, indicating the care with which the bread for allergic patients must be purchased or made. Ry-Krisp made in America is of pure rye. Most Scandinavian knäckebröd or pure rye hardtack is made of pure rye flour, but at times is dusted with wheat flour. A common use of rye is in the making of whiskey.

Oats (avena sativa) was first mentioned in Roman writings as being used by the Germans. Since it lacks gliadin, it cannot be leavened into bread. It is used in gruels, cakes, mush, certain crackers, cookies, and muffins.

Barley (hordeum distichon) probably was the first cereal to be used by man, as recorded by Egyptians. Its principal present use is in the making of malt. The barley is allowed to sprout or germinate so that diastatic enzymes are formed. These convert starch into sugar in the manufacture of beer and ale and the sugar is then converted into alcohol by yeast. *Beer, ale, stout, and porter* are thus made with malt of barley, and at times, of wheat, rice and corn. Some *whiskey and gin* are made with barley. Pearl barley is used as a breakfast food and in soups and broths. The breakfast foods containing barley are listed on page 229.

Rice (oryza sativa) was used in China 3000 years B.C. and is the important food of one-third of the world's populace today. It is raised in flooded warm areas extensively in Asia, and in California, Texas, the Carolinas and in similar regions in the United States. Unpolished rice is usually used in the Orient. Polishing, in this country, removes the husk and with it most of the vitamins A and B. Rice flour makes poor bread because of its lack of gliadin. Vermicelli or macaroni can be made of pure rice flour.

"Sake" in Japan is a beer made from rice. Various products containing rice are listed on page 232. Because of the large content of vitamin B in rice polishings, they are used as such or in concentrates in various vitamin preparations.

Wild rice (zizania aquatica) is similar to ordinary rice but biologically different. It was a food of the native Indians. It grows on a tall grass in swampy borders of lakes, streams, and rivers from Canada down the Mississippi Valley and is eaten frequently here in America.

Corn (*zea mays*) has been grown in the Americas for food probably a thousand years, being generally used by the Indians when Europeans first arrived. Low in gliadin, corn meal makes a crumbly bread. It is used in varying proportions and with different ingredients in corn pone, spoon bread, ash cake, batter bread, griddle, and pan cakes. Corn meal is the main ingredient in most tamales and tortillas, enchilades, Italian polenta, and in other Mexican dishes. *Wheat, however, is usually in these products.* Corn meal, ground between stones, keeps poorly because of the corn germ which contains fat. Processed corn meal, freed from the germ, dried in a kiln and rolled at a high temperature between rollers, spoils less readily and can be mixed with other flours for baking. White and yellow corn meals are made. A special species of Indian corn with much endosperm in hard kernels is used for popcorn. Corn oil is obtained by pressing the germ. It is used for salad oil, Mazola oil being of this kind, and it also is used in soaps, paints and salad dressings. Cornstarch is used in puddings, sauces, gravies, and soups and especially in the laundry. A vegetable gum, dextrin, and British gum is used on postage stamps, envelopes and in the finishing of many textiles. Corn syrup or commercial glucose is made from cornstarch. Karo is the usual product sold, though corn glucose is used in many candies, jellies, preserves, maple syrups, and other sweetened products. Corn is also used to make whiskey and some beer. A list of products containing corn is found on page 232.

Sorghum (sorghum vulgare) is not closely allied to corn. It is a grain from a grass similar to Johnson or barnyard grass. One species is used to make sorghum molasses and another for grain which is ground to make pan cakes, puddings, or with other flours is made into bread in the southern states.

Cane Sugar (saccharum officinarum), a member of the grass family, was first grown in Bengal, eaten in Indio China, the Malay States, Africa, and in Europe in the eighth century. It was brought to America by Columbus, and today is grown in all warm, moist areas in the world. In the United States, a yearly average of 94 pounds per person is used. The question of allergy to cane sugar is unsettled. The amount of allergen from the original cane itself is so infinitesimal, even if present, that sensitization to it or any other possible ingredient in purified cane sugar is hardly conceivable. Many people attribute symptoms to sugar, whereas other ingredients in desserts, cake, or candy, such as chocolate, milk, wheat, nuts, or fruit are responsible. As Vaughan states, sugar might act as a hapten and cause allergy as described on page 26. Allergy to the unpurified molasses may occur, though no records are published. Most commercial molasses contains corn glucose. There is some evidence that patients may be allergic to cane sugar and not to beet sugar or corn glucose. Those sensitive to beet sugar pollen or to beets might be sensitive to *beet sugar* if allergens in such sugar actually exist.

Millet is another cereal grain used as a food in Asia and in animal feeds in this country.

Bamboo (bambusa) is another grass, the young shoots of which are used for food in the Orient and by the Chinese here in America. The grains or seeds of the bamboo are not used as food.

OTHER CARBOHYDRATE-RICH FOODS

White potato (solanum tuberosum) is closely related to the tomato, red and green pepper, and eggplant. A native of Chile and Peru, it was brought to Europe by Raleigh and then to the American colonies. The potato forms on an underground stem as a growth or tuber. The sweet potato is different botanically and is a fleshy root. The white potato apparently is a growth due to irritation of specific ground fungi on the terminal bud of the stem. This food produces various allergic manifestations, but less frequently than do cereal grains. At times, potato and tomato allergy occur in one patient. Often apparent allergy to potato is due to foods such as butter, milk, wheat, cottonseed oil, pepper, etc., with which the potato is cooked. Potato flour, combined with rice, rye or with egg alone and other ingredients, make satisfactory cakes, muffins, and cookies. It may be used as a thickening or in place of cornstarch or in various bakery and culinary recipes. Potato chips are cooked in various vegetable oils, especially cottonseed oil to which allergy may exist. Potato syrup and sugar are also used in Europe.

Sweet potato (*ipomoea batatas*) is a member of the morning glory family and is the fleshy root. It is eaten as are white potatoes. Candied, baked sweet potato is popular. Glucose and alcohol are

5

derived products. Its flour is used in the Orient. *Yam* is a watery sweet potato grown in the southern states and is different from the Oriental yam which is a member of the lily family.

Tapioca (manihot utilissima) is a starch from the cassava or manioc obtained from the roots of the tree. Many varieties are grown in Equatorial South America, Central America, Africa, India, and the East Indies, where it is a common food. In America it is sold as pearl, granulated, flaked tapioca or as a flour. It is of special value in cereal-free elimination diets. The cassava starch is used in yeast cakes and as a laundry starch.

Sago (metroxylon sagu) is obtained from the pith of the sago palm in the East Indies which is engorged with starch just before the palm bears fruit at the age of ten to fifteen years. Other species such as læve and rumphii also yield sago.

Arrowroot (maranta arundinacea) is a starch made from the plant's root or rhizome grown in Brazil, West Indies, Florida, Georgia, Mississippi, East Indies, South Africa, and Mexico. It is used in bakery products, puddings, and as a thickener in soup, broths, and milk.

Florida arrowroot, Coontie, or Indian bread-root (zamia integrifolia) comes from the pith of the trunk and roots of the palm. This starch may be used like arrowroot above.

Taro, kalo (colocasia antiquorum esculenta) is grown in many varieties in the Hawaiian Islands, Tahiti, Japan, East and West Indies as an important source of starch. Poi is a fermented paste pounded from the roots. The roots may be eaten as potatoes. The cooked leaves are used as a palatable vegetable.

Breadfruit (artocarpus communis) belongs to the mulberry to which figs and hops belong. It was native in the South Sea Islands and is a prolific source of nourishment for eight months of the year. The fruit is 6 to 8 inches in diameter. The edible part lies between the thin skin and the small core. It is white and resembles new bread in texture. When baked or roasted, it thickens and tastes like sweet potato. This food might be of value to the allergic patient here in America.

Buckwheat (fagopyrum esculentum) is related to rhubarb, the flour coming from grinding the large seeds. A native of Europe and Asia, it was raised by Chinese a thousand years ago. It grows on poor soil in many areas, even in high altitudes. Since the seed resembles the beech nut, its name is derived from the German buchweizen, or beech wheat. The pure flour may be used for cakes and bread. Commercial flour is usually mixed with other flours. Jews make a pure buckwheat soup called Kasha.

Flaxseed (linaceæ) comes from flax, the fiber of which has been used to make cloth since Egyptian time. The seeds were eaten by Greeks and Romans. It still is used in Uncle Sam's Breakfast Food, and especially in stock feed, chicken mashes and feeds. Flaxseed tea and poultices have been used medicinally for many years. It is used as a hair set, though karaya gum is preferred. Allergy may be severe, often associated with a large scratch reaction. *Linseed* oil is made from flaxseed and is used in paints, varnishes, in furniture and floor oils and polishes, and in printer's and lithographer's inks. Linoleum, oilcloth, oilskin coats, and other articles are made with it. It may also be in depilatories and hair tonics.

Flours made from soy and lima beans, from banana, sweet potatoes and chestnut will be discussed under vegetables, fruits, and nuts.

DAIRY PRODUCTS

Milk.—*Milks from different animals,* including the cow, goat, mare, sheep, ass, camel, and from other animals are used in varying parts of the world. Human milk from wet nurses or in cans is also used in pediatrics. In America and Europe, cows' milk and, secondly, goat's milk are most frequently used. Clinical and experimental evidence indicates that the lactalbumins in the wheys of different milks contain dissimilar protein allergens and that the caseins of such milks are probably identical. Lactalbumin allergy is more frequent than casein allergy which probably explains why patients sensitive to cow's milk may tolerate goat's milk. Recent work, however, indicates that allergens common to the lactalbumins of several milks may exist, producing allergy from all such milks. The effect of pasteurization, boiling, superheating, and drying of milk on its allergenic activity has been discussed on page 60. Mare, sheep, and camel milks are used as such or in cheeses in southern Europe, Asia, Africa, and other countries where cows and goats are not common.

Though milk is an important food, especially in infancy, it is not essential at any age for proper nutrition. Here in America, the dairy and milk dispensing interests have so stressed the value of milk that the opinion unfortunately is widely held that 1 quart or more of milk a day is necessary for young children and adolescents and that 1 pint or more is important for adults. Stress on such quantities because of the calcium content is unnecessary. If milk is entirely omitted, calcium carbonate, gluconate or other salt given daily, (see page 146) together with a proper amount of other foods, will meet the accepted daily requirement of 1 gram of available calcium. Many adults give a history of taking no

milk or additional calcium for many years with no evident deple-
tion in calcium in their bones.   Indeed, many such milk-sensitive
people have excellent physiques and perfect teeth, often with no
decay.   The protein content of milk can be replaced by equal
amounts of protein in meat, fowl, fish, legumes, and eggs.   The
vitamin content of milk can readily be supplied by those in other
foods or by the vitamins themselves.   The great majority of the
world's population, of course, drink little or no milk of any type
after they are weaned.   Moreover, the importance of calcium in
the prevention of tooth decay is very doubtful, in spite of advertise-
ments and certain dentists.   Thus, though milk is a very excellent
food for all ages, particularly for infants and children, it is not
essential and can be entirely eliminated without nutritional damage, providing the proper amount of protein, fats, calories, vitamins, and minerals, especially calcium, are contained in the diet
recommended by the physician or dietitian cognizant of the carbohydrate, protein, fat, mineral, and vitamin content of foods.
As examples of such milk-free diets, all the menus for the elimination diets and the diets recommended for milk sensitive infants
and young children in this book are available.   The diet from
which milk alone is excluded is discussed on page 199.

*Since the milk, serum, meat, skin, and hair of an animal such as
the cow contain a small amount of identical allergens and other
entirely dissimilar and specific ones, certain patients may become
sensitive to the milk, meat, and emanations, originally being sensitized
to only one.*   Thus, some patients sensitive to cow's milk are also
allergic to the meat of beef or its organ products and to cattle
dander.   Such sensitization to horse meat, dander, and serum is
noted on pages 73 and 105

Cow milk allergy occurs in 20 to 30 per cent of all food sensitive
individuals.   As in other food sensitive patients, good scratch
reactions may only occur when marked or immediate manifestations arise.   Many clinically sensitive patients fail to give such
skin tests.   Milk allergy tends to run through several generations
of certain families, as noted on page 20.   Overfeeding and the
forcing of milk probably sensitizes many infants, children and even
adults.   *Aversion for milk and anorexia or lack of appetite not
infrequently* are due to milk or other food allergy.   A gradual improvement of appetite and increase in weight often occurs with the
elimination of allergenic foods among which milk is extremely
frequent.   Thus, milk sensitive children who have been spoon fed,
forced to eat with the aid of promises and stories, may develop
good appetites and eat with relish at and between meals when
such foods are entirely excluded.

Allergy may develop to allergens which pass from the blood into the milk. Thus, allergens of various foods eaten by the mother may occur in her milk. Their amounts, it is true, are nearly infinitesimal but sufficient to cause symptoms in the sensitized infant. In the same way, allergens from grasses, weeds and their pollens, flaxseed, cottonseed meal, peanuts, grains, or other foods, may occur in cow's milk. Thus, milk from a cow at one season and not at another may cause symptoms in the allergic individual. The presence of various pollens in honey is suggested by this as noted on page 98.

Allergy to milk as to other foods varies in degree. Very sensitive patients cannot take a small amount of butter which contains a minute amount of milk. Moderately sensitive patients may take moderate amounts of butter or cream but no definite amounts of milk. They may also take denaturized, heated, canned, or dried milk in varying amounts. Patients sensitive only to lactalbumin may eat various cheeses as discussed below. Mild milk allergy may produce subclinical slight symptoms which make the patient feel under par or slightly ill without actual or obvious symptoms. Various foods which contain milk are listed on page 229.

Goat's milk, as already stated, produces allergy in many patients sensitive to cow's milk, especially when casein allergy exists. All that has been written above concerning cow's milk applies to goat's milk, though the latter is used in small amounts here in America. If goat's milk is used, it must be adequately pasteurized to prevent transmission of infections, including diphtheria, streptococcal infections, undulant fever, tuberculosis and others. Canned goat's milk is sold by the Goat Milk Products Company of Los Angeles. Other substitutes for cow's milk especially for infant feeding are discussed on page 199.

Cream and Butter.—It is important to realize that *cream and butter contain milk proteins and other allergens.* Fifty to 80 per cent of cream as sold consists of milk according to its consistency. Butter contains a minimum of 0.6 per cent of milk curd or casein and up to 1.2 per cent according to the thoroughness with which the butter granules are washed with pure water after the buttermilk is drained off. A trace of lactalbumin and other milk proteins is also present. This small amount of milk allergens is sufficient to produce severe allergy in patients very allergic to milk, especially if casein allergy is present. This was illustrated in the case of a young girl who had severe attacks of asthma with fever up to 104°, delirium for six to fourteen hours, and vomiting for several hours, due to food allergy, especially from milk. After being off of milk in every form for one year, a teaspoonful of butter was given and in three hours the above symptoms occurred with dramatic severity. Various butter substitutes are listed on page 156. Butter is colored generally with 2 ounces of a yellow fluid made from annatto seeds to every 1000 pounds of butter or with other coloring matter. No study has ever been made concerning possible allergy to this seed.

Oleomargarines contain various vegetable and animal fats and milk protein. Most of these are churned in milk or cream and contain up to 2 per cent milk casein. Annatto or other coloring and salt are added. Allergy may exist to the allergens in any of the fats as well as to the milk allergens. Their use, therefore, is contraindicated in milk sensitive patients and in those sensitive to the specific fat incorporated in the oleomargarine. Some butter substitutes contain no milk products. Nuspread is made with a hydrogenated cottonseed oil, colored light yellow and flavored with butyric acid. Another similar product made of hydrogenated sesame oil, artificial color and flavor can be obtained from Calden & Bray, Piedmont Ave., Oakland, Calif.

Cheese.—Cheese contains milk proteins, usually casein with minute amounts of lactalbumin. Patients only sensitive to the latter protein may be able to take the cheeses made nearly exclusively of casein. However, those exceedingly sensitive to lactalbumin might react to the trace of this allergen in practically all cheeses and especially to those cheeses which contain larger amounts of whey or lactalbumin such as cottage, cream, or buttermilk cheese, Neufchatel, Gervais, Scandinavian or Danish mysost cheeses. Vaughan has listed the following cheeses made of cow's milk:

American Cheese	Floedoest	Pineapple
Appetitost	Gammelost	Pont L'Eveque
Bondost	Gervais	Port du Salut
Brick	Gorgonzola	Pennsylvania Pot
Brie	Gouda	Provolone
Buttermilk	Goya	Rabbit
Caciocavallo	Gruyere	Rat
California Jack	Hand	Sage
Camembert	Koesher Gouda	Sap Sago
Cheddar	Leyden	Sbrinz
Cheshire	Liederkranz	Smearcase
Cottage	Limburger	(Schmierkase)
Cream	Lodigiano	Sorrento
D'Isigny	Munster	Stilton
Dunlop	Mysost	Store
Edam	Neufchatel	Schweizer
Emmenthaler	Oka	Swiss
English Dairy	Parmesan	

Vaughan, The Practice of Allergy, St. Louis, C. V. Mosby Company, p. 419, 1939.

Goat's milk is used to make Gjedeost, a brown, sweet, strong flavored, Norwegian cheese. Gorgonzola and Montasio are, at times, made from goat's milk. Lipton's is made from goat's milk, flavored with spices and pepper. Sheep's milk is used in Roquefort cheese and in Italian cheeses such as Romano, Sardegna, Toscano, and Pecorino. Imitations made from cow's milk are also sold. Other animal milks, of course, are used to make various cheeses. Koumiss is fermented asses' or mares' milk.

Every area in the world has various local cheeses, with special names made with varying ingredients. Most cheese is fermented in its preparation with lactic acid bacilli. Thereafter, molds of varying types may be used to "ripen" the cheese and patients may become allergic to these various molds or fungi. Penicillia are used in Roquefort and Camembert cheese. Gammelort has so much fungus finally that the curd is nearly replaced. Other cheeses are flavored with spices such as sage, cloves, caraway, various herbs, pimento and other substances to which allergy may develop.

Egg.—Egg allergy, especially to its albumen in the white but also to the protein in the yolk, is very common and is responsible for many and often severe allergic manifestations. This allergy may be present at birth, apparently arising from sensitization in the uterus by egg eaten by the mother or through an inherited propensity to egg allergy. It may be extremely severe in degree at any time of life, especially in infancy and childhood and is often associated with a large scratch skin test. As all egg products are eliminated from the diet for several years, such skin reactions may disappear and tolerance for egg may arise. When egg allergy is active, sensitization to the albumen and the yolk is usually present. Moreover, it is practically impossible to separate yolks so that every trace of albumen is absent. Therefore, the elimination of the white, as well as the yolk, should be insisted upon in egg sensitive patients.

Egg is used in the manufacture of most ice creams and many sherbets, mousses, and water ices. The commercial ice cream and dessert powders may contain powdered egg, milk, and other ingredients. Egg, also, is in most cakes, cookies, many breads, especially whole wheat bread, French toast, pastries, muffins, frostings, icings, meringues, custards, puddings, waffles, hot and griddle cakes, cream sauces, desserts, prune and other whips, salad dressings and mayonnaise. Macaroni, spaghetti, noodles, pastes, batters, meat molds, preserved meats, certain sausages, beef juices, meat jellies, and some cake and pancake flours often contain egg.

Egg is in many candies, especially "filled" ones, in chocolate and other "bar" confections, in fondants, creams, nougats, and many marshmallows.   Egg is often rubbed over buns, bread, and pretzels to produce a glaze.   Breads may be sprayed with egg or milk to produce a sheen and crust.   Some baking powders (not Royal, K–C, Schillings, or Calumet) contain minute amounts of egg. Ovaltine, Ovomalt, and similar products consist of dried egg, milk and chocolate.   Soups, coffee, and wines are frequently cleared with egg albumen.   Chefs like to soak chicken, fritters, and other food in egg before cooking and they use egg in many other recipes, often in small amounts.   Certain pharmaceutical emulsions and other medical preparations, such as some nose drops, contain egg. Therefore, the egg sensitive patient must keep all these possibilities in mind and must never take any food whose absolutely accurate content is not known.

Egg yolk is used by furriers in dressing some skins, in tanning and preparing some glove leather.   Egg albumen is used in photography as a film emulsion and in printing cotton and textile fabrics which might produce contact eczema in very sensitive patients.

The use of other eggs as of ducks or turkeys by hen egg allergic patients is not advisable since the albumens of eggs of various birds are similar antigenically.   There probably are group allergens and species specific allergens for various eggs, as discussed on page 62 for other allergens.   Further experimental study of the relationship of the various allergens in eggs of different birds and of their relationship to the allergens in the flesh, blood, and other tissues of such birds is important.   Some patients sensitive to egg are also sensitive to the feather and meat allergens, but this is not the rule.

MEATS

Allergy to the meat and organ tissues of the mammalian animals occurs but less frequently than to milk, egg, cereal grains, fish, and certain other foods.   Through immunological animal experimentation, it has been shown that similar allergens exist in the tissues of closely related animals.   As with other groups of foods such as cereal grains, milks, and eggs from biologically related animals, certain allergens in the closely related meats probably are identical and others may be specific for each animal.   Thus allergy may occur in varying degrees to all meats or specifically to only one, such as beef or pork.   Again a patient may be allergic to the meat, liver, kidney, brains, or other edible tissues of the same animal or only to one or two of them. Much more study in the laboratory of the various allergens in such mammalian tissues and of their interrelationships is urgently needed. Whether the foods fed to such animals as corn, peanuts, various grains, or beet tops, influence the allergic reactivity of the meats needs experimental study. The final determination of the patient's reactivity to such meats and tissues, as in all food allergies, must depend on actual diet trial, the food in question being given to the symptom-free patient for a number of days. Even with such diet trial, potential or very mild allergy may not be demonstrable. Moreover, reactions to various meats may be due to the condiments, gravies, or fats cooked or served with the meats.

Beef causes various allergic manifestations in a small number of patients. Vaughan estimates that about 4 per cent of beef allergies are associated with cow's milk allergy though the sensitization may be to one or the other food alone. One patient was allergic to beef, lamb, and pork and could take milk with no difficulty. Veal coming from the baby steer or cow should be similar to beef. However, an occasional patient has a specific allergy to veal alone as reported by Kern.

Lamb causes less allergy than beef and pork and consequently has been used in my elimination diets and in other trial diets.

Pork causes more allergy than either beef or lamb, the manifestations at times being severe in type. A physician who had a rash from pork all her life could not take lard or even a 1 grain thyroid pill of pork origin without such a rash. At times such allergics can eat ham and especially bacon, probably due to the changed reactivity of the pork protein by the smoking and processing of the pork. Bacon, moreover, usually contains a comparatively small amount of meat and is denaturized by the high temperature of frying. Various allergens which accumulate in ham or bacon during their processing and curing from smoke might in the rare individual produce allergic reactivity. Foods and condiments used in the cooking of hams and gravies are discussed below.

Horse meat is used in Europe and to a varying extent in other countries. Its use in dog food here in America makes possible its accidental human consumption. As discussed on page 105, a group sensitization to such meat, horse dander, and horse serum may exist. Sensitization to one may create allergy to all. Mare's milk, moreover, is used at times, especially in Russia, and children fed with it may become allergic to horse serum. *Goat* meat when eaten may establish allergy.

Rabbit, squirrel, and other rodentia meats may cause allergy in susceptible patients. Reindeer and other *deer* meat must be remembered as a more or less frequent food. Other mammalia, such as bears, buffalo, and various rodents, are eaten in different world areas and may cause allergy. Such meats of mammalian animals which do not belong to the Bovidæ, as shown on page 226, might be of value to the occasional patient who cannot take beef, lamb, or pork.

Liver allergy, producing various manifestations, may exist along with or independent of allergy to the meat. Thus asthma developed in one patient from beef or lamb liver and from the liver extract given for anemia but not from beef or lamb meat or, interestingly, from chicken's liver. Such liver allergy must be remembered because of the important use of liver extracts for anemia and for vitamin deficiencies. Specific allergy to other organ tissues, especially to thyroid, pancreas, pituitary, and adrenal is discussed when drug and hormonal allergies are described below.

Gelatin.—*Gelatin, like glue, is made from hides, horns, connective tissue, and cartilage of various animals.* It is used in cooking, bouillon tablets, in medicinal capsules, and in the industries. Gelatin fails to produce experimental anaphylaxis in animals. Wells attributed this to the absence of the amino-acids tryptophane and tyrosin which may be necessary for the development of allergy. Or, possibly, the arrangement of the carbon atoms in a chain, rather than a ring in the molecule, may prevent allergic reactivity. Clinically, occasional evidence of allergy to gelatin arises. This may be due to traces of the beef or other animal tissue used in the making of gelatin.

Fowl.—The flesh of many *tame and game birds* is eaten, those most commonly used, such as chicken and duck, causing the most allergy. As Vaughan notes, the members of this bird family, including chicken, wild and tame ducks, goose, turkey, pheasant, squab, quail, guinea and sage hen, doves, pigeon, snipe, and many others are rather distantly related. Thus, allergy to one is rarely associated with allergy to the others. However, sensitization to one species of chicken or duck usually means allergy to all species. The effect of the predominate feed on the allergenic activity of the flesh of these various birds is a problem which needs study as noted on page 69.

Sensitization to the meat of a bird may be accompanied with allergy to the bird's feathers and emanations; or such feather allergy may be absent as is true with meats and emanations of

animals discussed on page 62.   Group and specific allergens exist
in the feathers of all types of birds.   The more closely related
species probably have more common group allergens.

As with meats, the allergic patient who is on an elimination or
specified diet must not eat fowl which has been rubbed with butter,
oil, or garnished or basted with any spices, condiments, or any
food preparation which has not been ordered and allowed by the
physician.   This care is also imperative in regard to stuffing or
other foods cooked in or with the fowl.   It is probable that some
patients are so sensitive to wheat, corn, or spices that when used
in the stuffing, allergens from such foods permeate the flesh or
adhere to the meat through proximity to the dressing and cause
symptoms when the meat is eaten.   Knowledge of all ingredients
in the gravies served with fowl also is essential.   Drippings from
the roasting fowl, of course, contain food allergens as of butter,
flour, oil, or garnishings rubbed on the bird or cooked therewith.
If such foods have not been allowed, the gravies should not be used.
Neither should spices nor pepper be incorporated unless specifically
ordered by the physician.

True Fishes (Vertebrates).—All the edible fishes except eels
have fins.   As will be seen from the classification of fishes on page
225, they belong to many different families and genuses.   As
Vaughan states, the evidence from skin testing and clinical study
of patient's actual allergies to fishes indicates that *sensitization
usually exists to several or many fishes in different families but not
necessarily to the fishes of all genuses and families.*   Indeed, specific
allergy to one fish with apparent tolerance to all others may occur.
Such crossed sensitizations are infrequently associated with allergy
to various shell fishes, though they may occur simultaneously.
That the same species of fish may have different names in different
areas must be remembered.   This is especially true of the sardine.
Testing is probably advisable with the allergens of one or two of
the representatives of the important families of fishes.   And the
testing with allergens of individual fishes which are commonly
eaten, especially if suspected by history, should be done.   As with
all food allergies, skin tests may be negative when clinical allergy
is present.   This seems less frequent than with milk, vegetable,
or fruit allergies; in fact, some of our largest skin reactions occur
to fish allergens.

These large scratch skin reactions are often associated with a
marked degree of clinical allergy.   The symptoms, be they asthma,
cutaneous, or gastro-intestinal manifestations often occur soon
after the eating of the fish, even a minute trace thereof.   The

inhalation of the fish allergens from fish cooking in a distant kitchen, or as Vaughan describes, from the eating of butter in which fish allergens have gathered from the air filled with allergens from fish in the same refrigerator may be sufficient to cause the allergic manifestation.   Such marked allergy and large skin reactions again indicate the importance of testing patients with the scratch method and only with the intradermal method when negative scratch tests are obtained.   (See page 24.)

The problem of group allergens and species specific allergens again arises as discussed concerning other foods on page 62.   Laboratory experimentation is urgently needed to understand the intricacies of such relationships and many other problems in the allergic field.   It may be that fishes and other foods eventually will be classified according to their content of group specific allergens and not by their biological relationship based on outward and structural characteristics.

Cod-liver oil, as noted by Balyeat and Bowen and by many other allergists, causes allergic rashes, asthma, or gastro-intestinal symptoms in sensitized patients, especially children.   This sensitivity gradually develops from the continued administration, or in some instances through an inherited specific propensity.   Some thirty species of fish, all members of the Gadies family, may be used to make U.S.P. cod-liver oil.   Such oil is especially rich in vitamin D.

Other fish oils are used because of their vitamin content in medical therapy.   Halibut-liver oil is rich in vitamin A, containing less vitamin D than does cod-liver oil.   Shark oil contains much vitamin D and other fishes, as noted above, contain these vitamins.

Caviar is usually sturgeon roe or eggs.   In America, the eggs of sturgeons, carp, shad, spoonbill, lake herring, and other fish are used for roe.   Thus, allergy may exist to one kind of roe and not to another.

The incorporation of small amounts of fish or fish oils in various foods, recipes, mixed foods, and sauces, and as adulterations in certain food oils must be remembered.   Vaughan notes the small amount of fish which is in some catsups.

Glue allergy is not especially common, but may be extremely severe.   It should be used in the routine testing of patients, especially those suffering with inhalant allergies.   It is often made from fish but is also made from bones, hides, and cartilages of any animal.   Some evidence indicates that glue allergy is always due to fish glue.   Such allergy is usually but not necessarily associated with allergy to the meats of fishes.   Extremely severe and even fatal symptoms have been described by Duke and Stofer, Cooke and others to infinitesimal amounts of glue, even to that used in scratch testing. When hyposensitization therapy is given, extremely dilute solutions must be injected, one case of the writer's being *given first a 1 to 500,000,000 dilution* with a very careful increase over a period of four years. His generalized and severe dermatitis was gradually controlled. Such inhalant allergy to glue is discussed on page 47.

Glue is used by cabinet workers, carpenters, on envelope flaps, in the making of pads and books, on sandpaper and matches, tablets, gummed paper, courtplaster, in sizing cloth, paper and carpets, in gelatin, jellies, isinglass, combs, buttons, mucilages, and pastes. The dust of furniture and books in homes, offices, drafting rooms, libraries contain varying amounts of glue. Severe reactions from the absorption from the glue used on the inner sole of shoes have been reported. The licking of stamps and labels may cause severe reactions in the lips and mouth or on distant tissues. Most stamps, however, are treated with a vegetable glue, as noted on page 47.

Shell Fishes (Invertebrates).—Some of the most severe clinical allergies develop to shell fish. Group allergies tend to develop to members of the same class or the allergy may be very specific, limited to one shell fish. Skin reactions by the scratch test usually are large. Sensitization may also occur to several distantly related shell fish as to those of the Gastropoda and Crustacea as tabulated on page 224.

The *abalone* is a large snail which lives on rocks in the ocean, especially in California. The mussel is cooked as such or in chowder. The *snail* is another edible Gastropoda. It is commonly eaten in Europe, especially in Paris, and tastes and looks like a shrimp.

Mussels, oysters, scallops, and clams are bivalve shell fish, belonging to the class Pelecypoda. All may produce allergy, especially those which are eaten most frequently in a given locality. Severe sensitizations with marked skin reactions may develop to these food allergens.

Squid is another mollusca, a small type of cuttle fish, eaten especially in the Mediterranean area. The shell is rudimentary, being a pen-shaped internal structure. It is usually cooked with egg, fried in oil and served with condiments and other foods.

Crab, lobster, crayfish, shrimp, and prawns are arthropods with skeletons outside, rather than inside their bodies. Group sensitizations are the rule though individual specific allergy may exist or predominate.   Allergy to one or all may be associated with allergy to the other shell fish such as oysters or clams and less often with allergy to the true (fin) fish.   That the type of food these shell fish consume may influence their allergenicity is indicated by Kern's observation that a patient was allergic to lobsters north of Cape Cod and not from the southern coast.   Similar effects from feeds in milk have been noted on page 69.

Amphibia and Reptiles.—*Frog legs* are eaten with increasing frequency and turtle meat is used in soups.   These animals are distantly related to others and might be prescribed, especially when milk, egg, or fish allergies are present.   Mock turtle soup contains no turtle but is made from meats, vegetables, spices, and other flavors.

Snake meat is eaten in certain areas of the world.   Here in America rattlesnake meat is occasionally eaten in the open areas and may be obtained in cans, according to Vaughan.

VEGETABLES

Certain vegetables tend to produce allergy more frequently than do others, though instances of allergy to practically all vegetables are not lacking.   Thus, allergy is especially likely to occur to lettuce, spinach, tomato, the various legumes, members of the cabbage group, onion and garlic.   Vaughan described sensitizations to related species of vegetables as to other types of food belonging to the same genus.   Though such group sensitizations are not the rule, they must be suspected, especially if a marked specific allergy to one vegetable exists.   Alvarez especially has stressed the necessity of realizing that indigestion may arise from irritants in vegetables and from organic causes such as gall bladder disease, peptic ulcer, appendicitis or other constitutional disease.   Such symptoms must not be attributed to food allergy.   This was discussed on page 109.   Allergy may exist to several distantly related vegetables and some rare patients are allergic to practically all vegetables.   When this occurs, allergy to all fruits may also exist, necessitating adequate supplemental vitamin therapy and careful attempted hyposensitization with all important vegetable and fruit allergens, as discussed on page 61.   The varying denaturizing effect of heat on vegetables must be remembered.

Onion (allium cepa) and **garlic** (allium sativum) belong to the family Liliaceæ and are productive of frequent and often severe allergy.   It is probably more common when these foods have been eaten in large or frequent amounts and particularly in the raw state. In the colder areas of this and other countries, onions may be eaten raw as are apples. The eating of small green onions is common. One patient became so allergic that the eating of two olives dipped in oil flavored with garlic produced dizziness, exhaustion even to collapse with nausea and vomiting. These foods are so frequently used as flavors in meats, fowl, fish, soups, salads, pickles, sausages, sauces, catsups, and other recipes, often in minute indiscernible amounts, that the patient must always be analytical of any flavored or mixed foods, especially soups, sauces, meat, fowl and fish preparations. Wild onion and garlic eaten by cows flavor their milk, indicating possible allergy from such milk and butter. As with other food allergies, all degrees of susceptibility exist so that traces of these foods may not produce allergy in one patient and may result in extreme symptoms in another.

Leek (allium porrum) was used in Roman days, originating possibly in Switzerland. The pungent odor and taste are decreased with cooking. It is used, especially in France, as is asparagus. The leaves are incorporated in soups, salads, and other recipes for their flavor.

Chives (allium schocnoprasum) came from Syria and are grown in Europe and America. The small red button is used to flavor soups, salads, meats, and stews.

Asparagus (asparagus officinalis) also belongs to Liliaceæ but to a different genus than the above vegetables and probably originated in the Caucasian region, being used in the early Christian era. The rapidly growing sprout from the root is eaten, being white when covered by the ground, becoming green above the ground. In Europe, the roasted seeds are used as a substitute for coffee and the root is made into a fermented drink. Vaughan mentions *yucca*, or Spanish bayonet, which is indigenous in the dry Southwest. The cluster fruit has a thick tender covering which, when cooked, is palatable.

The Beet Family (Chenopodiaceæ).—The *beet* (beta vulgaris) has been eaten since the 16th century. The young green leaves, boiled and seasoned, are eaten as greens. The esculent enlarged root is favored as a vegetable either hot, cold in salads, canned, or preserved with spices and vinegar—allergy to all of which must be remembered as a possibility.

The sugar beet first used as a source of cooking sugar in about 1800 now furnishes a large amount of the world's supply. Allergy to beet and cane sugar might exist and be distinct from each other, as noted on page 64.

Chard, sea kale (beta cycla) first developed in Africa and was used by Greeks and Romans. The leaf is made into salads or may be cooked as greens. The stem and moderately fleshy root from which the beet was developed may be eaten as such.

Spinach (spinacia oleracea), a member of Chenopodiaceæ, belongs to a different genus than do beet and chard. Used first in the 14th century in Europe, it originated in southwestern Asia. It is an important leaf vegetable, containing several important vitamins. (See note, page 203.) Vaughan notes that New Zealand spinach and mountain spinach are not related to true spinach. *Orache* is an atriplex and is distantly related to ordinary spinach.

In discussing possible allergy to these foods, it must be remembered that the pollens of many weeds belonging to this family, including the atriplexes, goose foots, Russian thistle, pig weeds, pickle weed, and sugar beet are common causes of allergy.

The Cabbage or Mustard Family (Brassicaceæ).—The many vegetables described below are related botanically and clinical allergies to them indicate that there are probably group allergens present in all or many and specific allergens only found in individual ones. Marked allergy to one or two should bring others of this group under suspicion. They probably came from a common origin, having differentiated themselves according to climatic and soil influences. Different parts of these plants are eaten. Thus, the seed of the mustard, the leaves of the cabbage, the abortive flower of the Brussels sprouts, the enlarged stem of kohlrabi, and the large top root of the rutabaga and turnip are used as vegetables.

Cabbage and kale or cole (brassica oleracea) were used by the Egyptians, Greeks and Romans, the firm head cabbage having developed in more recent times. Kale has open growing leaves and is of many varieties. Its former name of cole or borecole has given rise to the term cole slaw. Slaw is the Danish word for salad. Cole slaw today and *sour kraut* are made of cabbage. Vinegar, salt and pepper are added to the former and yeast is used to ferment the latter.

Collards (brassica oleracea acephala), especially grown in the South, is a variety of kale, the leaves forming in tufts which are cooked for food. The young leaves of cabbage are also called collards.

Cauliflower (brassica oleracea var. botrytis) is a type of kale in which the flowers are exaggerated and leaves remain open. *Broccoli* is a non-heading plant and hardier than the cauliflower, the flowers being smaller and less compact.

Brussels sprouts (brassica oleracea var. gemmifera) were grown in Belgium in the 13th century. They are cabbage plants which develop small cabbage sprouts along the large stems of the plant.

Kohlrabi (brassica oleracea var. caulo-rapa) seems to have developed from a cross between cabbage and rape which is a type of turnip fed to stock. This name has arisen from kale which, as noted above, is a loose growing cabbage or rape. Kohlrabi is similar to a turnip but grows above the ground as a fleshy stem.

Mustard (brassica nigra), known since ancient times, is grown for the seed. In the western states, another variety is a rank-growing weed. The pungent taste of mustard results from the production of a volatile oil from the action of water and a specific enzyme on the mustard flower. This was discovered by a woman of Durham, England, accounting for the name "Durham mustard." Mustard, as used on the table, usually contains mustard, vinegar, water, and flour and possibly other condiments. The cooked leaves of white mustard are used as greens.

Radish (raphanus sativus) originated in China and was used by Egyptians and Greeks. It is related to the cabbage group of vegetables and is used as an hors-d'œuvre and a relish.

Water cress (radicula nasturtium-aquaticum) grows in soil overrun by shallow water. The leaves are used generally the world over as a salad.

Horseradish (radicula armoracia) is closely related to water cress and less so to the cabbage group. It originated in eastern Europe. Its white pungent root is grated, moistened with vinegar, and is used as a condiment for meats and in salads.

Legumes (Leguminosæ).—The various legumes are extensively used for food all over the world and allergies are quite frequent, often to many in this group and less frequently to specific ones. As with all food allergies, sensitizations to these foods may produce manifestations in various tissues as discussed in Chapter III. The high content of protein makes legumes important in nutrition. I agree with Vaughan that peanut most commonly produces allergy, often of a severe type and associated with good scratch reactions.

Lentils (lens ecculenta) were raised in ancient days by the Egyptians and Hebrews and are still used as food, especially in Europe.

Beans (phaseolus) constitute a most important widely used food. *Lima beans* originated in Brazil and are grown extensively

6

in the Americas. *Kidney beans* originated here in America and are grown in several species, the *haricot* in France, the *frijole* in Mexico, the *white, navy and red beans* in this country, and other varieties in other countries. The pod of the *string bean* is eaten before the beans mature. The Chinese eat the sprouts, especially of the Mung bean, before the leaves appear. Various flours are prepared from different beans, especially from the lima bean in California.

Soy [Soja] Beans (soja max) originated in China and has been used there, and recently here in America, as a food. Because of the high protein and fat and low starch content, and the presence of all important amino-acids, protein requirements can be met with these beans. Soy bean products low in starch are used in diabetic foods. The flour combined with lima bean or potato flours is incorporated with other ingredients to make cereal-free bakery products in the elimination diets. Ordinary soy and lima bean breads, however, contain wheat and often milk. It is also used in a special preparation as a substitute for milk in infant feeding, as described on page 183. The Chinese make a cheese from soy bean called tofa, a brown sauce called soy, and a soy bean milk from the flour mixed with water. They also utilize soy in noodles, meat recipes, and in other food.

Duke noted the definite tendency to soy bean allergy. Sensitization to other legumes was present in some of these patients. He listed the various food products which at times contain soy bean, again showing the importance of knowing all ingredients in commercially prepared foods of all types. Soy bean may be in certain cakes, bread, muffins, crackers, macaroni, noodles, breakfast, diabetic, and allergic foods, in confections, sausage, in some condensed milks and coffee substitutes. Much oil from soy beans is used in making many commercial products, such as paints, varnishes, lubricants, linoleum, water-proof goods, soaps, celluloid, and printer's ink.

Peas (pisum) have been grown and eaten since earliest history and are eaten green as a vegetable. The dried, split peas, because of the protein content are helpful in milk- and egg-free diets and may be used in a puree, as a drink, hot or cold, or in soups, as described on page 158. Whereas soy bean contains all amino-acids essential for humans, other legumes do not.

Peanuts (arachis hypogæa) originated in tropical America. They develop in the pod which has formed on the flower stalk which has gradually bent toward the ground and finally worked itself into the soil. Some call it the ground pea. It is not a nut.

Eaten as a food since the Civil War, it is now used in large amounts in the roasted state, in the pods or shelled, in candy, cakes or breads. Peanut butter is especially popular in America. The flour is used in bread, especially in Europe. Peanut oil, as such or to adulterate other salad oils, is in common use.

The Carrot Family (Umbelliferæ).—These foods thrive in the temperate areas. The leaves, stalks, roots, or seeds may be used in salads as vegetables, garnishes, flavors, or spices.

Carrots (daucus carota) originated in Europe and later were grown in Asia and India, in the Middle Ages. Only the wild plant was used by the Greeks. They may be eaten raw and especially cooked. Carrot marmalade is acceptable as described on page 249.

Celery (apium graveolens) grew first in Europe. In ancient days it was used as a medicine, the assumed rapid action of which possibly accounts for its name. The stalks and fleshy stem and root may be eaten raw or cooked, in salads, as vegetables, or in soups. The leaves may garnish food or are made into celery salt.

Parsnips (peucedanum sativum) came from Europe, formerly used as a medicine. The root has been eaten as a vegetable for several centuries.

Parsley (carum petroselinum) was indigenous in Europe and was eaten by Greeks and Romans, being used in England first in the 16th century. It is used as a seasoning to soups and to garnish foods. The wild "fool's parsley" is poisonous. The Hamburg tulip-rooted parsley is eaten and is about equal in size to a small parsnip.

Fennel (fœniculum vulgare) looks like asparagus. The leaves may be used to flavor sausage, the stalks may be used in salads, and the seeds to flavor candies and liquors.

Caraway seeds (carum carvi) are aromatic and as spices are used in bakery products, in candies and cooking. The essential oil is used in perfumes and soaps. The alcoholic beverage, kümmel, is distilled from the seeds. *Coriander seeds* and leaves (coriandrum sativum) have been used since ancient times as are caraway seeds. *Aniseed* (myrrhis odorata) has the same use. A liquor, anisette, is made from it. Oil of anise is a favorite flavor for candy, cake, cookies, gum, dentrifices, and mouth washes.

Dill (anethum graveolenes) was used in Roman times. The seeds flavor sausage and pickles. The leaves have a taste of mint or fennel.

The Potato Family (Solanaceæ).—The various members of this family used as foods are all related to white potato, already described on page 65.

Tomato (lycopersicum esculentum), as cultivated, originated in Central and South America, was taken to Europe and, about a hundred years ago, first used as a food in our country. The vitamin content and the flavor of the food have increased its popularity. It is used fresh in salads, or cooked as a vegetable. It is used in sauces and as flavors for soups and pastes, especially in Spanish or Mexican foods. Tomato juice in cans or bottles is a good beverage.

Peppers (capsicum annuum) originated in the Americas, and the many varieties are now grown all over the world. Red pepper, *cayenne pepper, paprika* and *tobasco* all come from varieties of capsicum, while the black and white peppers come from an entirely different plant. (See page 95.) The paprika producing variety has a mild flavor and is eaten as a fresh vegetable. The Mexican chile has a strong "hot" flavor, first originating in Chile. *Green peppers* are unripened red peppers. Peppers are used in catsup, tamales, and in many soups, salads and Mexican and Spanish foods.

Eggplant (solanum melongena) is somewhat egg shaped and grows like a berry on a plant. Originating probably in India, it has been eaten in Europe, Asia and China since the 7th or 8th century.

The Gourd Family (Cucurbitaceæ).—Allergies to all members of this group and to individual members occur as with other closely related foods.

Squash, Pumpkin, Gourd (cucurbita) grow on creeping vines and probably originated in America, being cultivated by the Indians. Several varieties of squash exist such as the Hubbard, *summer, Italian or crookneck* varieties. Many varieties of the pumpkin are grown in different world areas. Vegetable marrow is a species grown often in England. Gourds with hard coverings, unusual odd shapes and colors are much used for ornaments. The dried and cleaned shell of these species may be used for water and food containers.

Cucumbers (cucumis sativus) grew first in Asia at least three thousand years ago, being used increasingly ever since. Picked green, they are treated with vinegar and spices to make pickles. Dill pickles are preserved with brine and dill. (See page 83.) *Gherkin* is a cucumber found in Jamaica but other cucumbers used for pickling are also so named.

Watermelon (citrullus vulgaris), found first in Africa, has been largely cultivated in America.

Cantaloupe or muskmelon (cucumis melo) was first popular in the Renaissance.

Many new melons such as the *Cassaba, Persian,* and *Crenshaw melons* may produce specific or group allergies.

Rhubarb (rheum rhaponticum) and buckwheat (see page 66) are members of the Buckwheat family. Rhubarb first grew in Asia. It was used in Italy in the early 17th century, in England two hundred years later, and was eaten in America in the early 19th century. The oxalic acid content of the leaves makes them dangerous as foods.

Okra—Gumbo (hibiscus esculentus) is related to cotton and belongs to the Mallow family. It originated in Africa. Its long pods may be eaten especially in soups to which a mucilaginous character is imparted. Vaughan reports urticaria from handling okra and gastro-intestinal symptoms from eating it.

The Thistle Family (Compositæ).—This family is extremely large, containing 10,000 or more species, mostly herbs, but also some shrubs and tropical trees. Group or crossed sensitization may exist, especially in closely related species.

Lettuce (lactuca sativa) originated in Europe and Asia and was used by the Greeks, Romans and Persians. Head lettuce has been grown for four hundred years.

Salsify or Oyster Plant (tragopogon porrifolius) has a fleshy root with an oyster-like flavor. It is used in salads, boiled, fried, or used as a relish. It was first used in Europe in the 16th century.

Endive (cichorium endiva) originated in India, and was eaten by the Greeks and Romans. Its leaves are used in salads.

Chicory (cichorium) was first grown as a vegetable in the 16th century. The leaves are used in salads, the young roots are cooked as a vegetable and the older roots, dried and ground, for a coffee substitute or adulterant. A volatile oil due to roasting yields an aroma.

Artichoke (cynara cardunculus) is a large thistle-like plant cultivated for its flowering heads which grow on stems. The soft inner surface of the leaves and the heart or bore of the flower heads, when cooked, are favored as a salad or vegetable. The canned hearts are used likewise.

Jerusalem artichoke (helianthus tuberosus) belongs to the sunflower family, being indigenous in North America. The name, as Vaughan says, was corrupted from the Italian girasole, meaning sunflower. The root resembling the potato is sweetish, is low in calories, and may be boiled, pickled, or eaten uncooked.

Dandelion (taraxacum) is grown in Europe, especially in France, for its edible young leaves, used in salads or boiled as greens.

Fruit—Allergy may be very specific to individual fruits or to biologically related fruits such as the citrus fruits or may exist to allergens common to practically all fruits. For patients suspected of possible allergy to all fruits, the fruit-free elimination diets on page 171 are available. Certain patients can take cooked and not raw fruits. Some are sensitive to the skins and not to the meat of the fruit.

Citrus fruits (rutaceæ) probably originated from a common origin in southeastern Asia. The outside skin has developed from modified leaves which united and entirely enclosed the berry-like fruit. It is widely cultivated in warm areas where freezing temperatures are rare.

Orange (citrus sinensis) was first cultivated in Europe in the 16th century. It is raised extensively in the southern states, especially in Florida, Texas, Arizona and California.

Orange oil from the rind, especially from Sicily, is used in perfumes, soaps, and flavors. Allergy to a dye used on green fruit has produced allergic dermatitis on the hands. Contact allergy to orange oil, especially on the hands, is not uncommon, as noted on page 120.

Sugar Orange, Seville, sour, bitter or brigrande orange, was the first one brought to Spain by the Moors in the 8th century. Being bitter and sour, it is only used in marmalade or candied or glacéd peel or for its oil.

Orange blossoms flavor some drinks in South America. The pollen from the blossoms produces some allergy.

Tangerine (citrus nobilis var. deliciosa) is a small orange which originated in China.

Lemon (citrus limonia) was brought to Europe by the Arabs. It usually is picked green, ripening gradually, especially in hotter temperatures up to 100° F. The oil is pressed from the rind, especially in southern Europe. It is used as is orange oil and in lemon extracts.

Grapefruit, pomelo, shaddock (citrus grandis) these varieties have white or red pulp. This first originated in the South Pacific and Malay Islands. It was first grown in Florida in the 16th century. Its name arose because of its growth in clusters. Modern cultivation is mainly in America.

Lime (citrus aurantifolia) is moderately different from the lemon, being used in candies, beverages, and as a flavor.

Limequat is a hybrid of the kumquat and the lime.

Kumquat or Fortunella, raised especially in China and Japan, is about 1 inch in diameter. The whole fruit is eaten, it may be used in salads, in preserves, jellies or marmalade.

Citron (citrus medica), first grown in India, was taken to Arabia and Syria and finally to Rome. The rind is used in candies, preserves, cakes, and puddings. The oil of citronella comes from the sweet Ceylonese grass.

Bergamot (citrus bergamia) oil has been used since the 17th century in perfumes.

The Apple Family (Pomaceæ).—**Apple** (malus) grows in the cool areas of North America, Europe, and other countries in many thousand variations. It was raised by the Romans and even by the original inhabitants of Central Europe. Vaughan has observed patients sensitive to cider vinegar and uses as a substitute, white vinegar. (See page 90.) Pectin, used in jellies, comes from the skins or cores of apples or from the rind of citrus fruits, and is also in cranberries, currants, gooseberries, and quinces. Pectin is used in some gumdrops and Turkish paste. Apple butter is made of concentrated cooked apple flavored with cider or vinegar, sugar, and spices. An imitation contains cornstarch, citric acid and apple oil.

Crab apples (malus coronaria), one variety native in America and one in Siberia, have a sour acrid taste when raw. Jellies and preserves are made by cooking them. The edible apple in its many varieties came originally from hybrids of the crab apples.

Quince (cydonia) originated in southern Europe and western Asia. It is unpleasant to eat in the raw state. When cooked, desirable jellies and jams are made. It contains a large amount of pectin.

Pear (pyrus) first grew in Europe and western Asia and is widely grown in temperate and cool areas of the world. Allergy to pear, at times, is associated with allergy to apple and other members of this group.

The Plum Family (Drupaceæ).—*These so-called pit fruits are closely related.* Allergy may exist to several or to individual ones. Almond is included, the meat of the pit developing and being eaten in comparison to the other fruits. The pits of almonds, apricots, peaches, and cherries are ground, fermented and distilled to produce almond oil. Hydrocyanic acid, also, is a product which is destroyed by lime and copperas. Prussic acid poisoning has resulted from the ingestion of the meat in the pits of wild cherries, bitter almonds, and peaches. Most of these fruits are sold fresh, dried, or canned. The drying may be in the sun alone or in dehydrators. Sulphur is commonly added as a preservative.

Apricot (prunus armeniaca) was indigenous in Arabia, America, and western Asia. It was first cultivated in England in the 17th century, and is grown now in temperate regions of the world.

Peach (prunus persica) first grew in China from whence it was brought to Asia Minor, Greece and Rome and later to Europe. Its assumed origin in Persia accounts for the name peach. Vaughan states that 1000 varieties of peaches have been developed.

Nectarines have smooth skin and have developed by bud variations from peaches. They have been grown and eaten for four hundred years.

Almond (prunus amygdalus) originated in Asia and North America. It is similar to the pit fruits. The meat of the pit is eaten, the fleshy part being thin and tough. Almond oil is described above.

Plum (prunus) grows in many varieties in temperate areas and is known often by regional names. It has been eaten for at least two thousand years. *Prunes* are special varieties which are dried and sold without removing the pits.

Cherry (prunus avium) also developed in the Caucasus region from where it was taken to southern and then to northern Europe and America. There are many cultivated varieties which originated from prunus cirasus and avium of Europe. Sour cooking cherries came from the former. Hybrids of the two species also have developed. The varieties vary in color from black to red and yellow. *Maraschino cherries* originally were preserved in a liqueur distilled from the marasca cherry. Imitations are common.

The Mulberry Family (Moraceæ).—The breadfruit (see page 91) and **hops** (see page 97) belong to this family as do the two fruits below.

Mulberry (morus) grows on trees of several varieties. Silkworms in China and Japan feed on the white mulberry. The black mulberry originated in and around Persia and bears an edible fruit. Vaughan suggests that the fruit of the red mulberry, a native of North America, be eaten more by allergic patients. It may be taken raw or cooked with such fruits as apples or rhubarb.

Fig (ficus carica) originated in Syria and the nearby area in ancient times. Several varieties are now grown in the southern states, especially California. Vaughan points out that the fig is not a true fruit, but a fruit receptacle, inside of which is the fruit or seed. At the end of this fleshy receptacle is a small orifice or "eye" surrounded by minute flowers. A special wasp ⅛ inch long which develops in the wild Capri fig only can fertilize the fig. The Smyrna fig only has pistillate flowers and no stamens. The Capri figs, containing the wasps, must be hung in the Smyrna fig trees so that the pollen from the Capri figs can be carried by the wasps to fertilize the Smyrna figs. The wasp is unable to emerge from the eye of the Smyrna fig and dies and is gradually absorbed by the fruit. Fresh or dried figs are used as such and cooked in jams and other recipes.

The following four fruits are very important but not related botanically.

Pineapple (ananas sativus) originated in tropical America. It is widely cultivated in tropical countries, especially in Hawaii, Philippines, China, India, Java, and Africa. It is eaten fresh or canned. The juice is canned and widely used. Pineapple allergy is not uncommon.

Banana (musa) has grown in torrid zones even in prehistoric times. Many varieties of bananas are known. The overlapping and tall upright leaf stalks grow from the root and from the trunk of the tree. With each harvest, this trunk is cut down and a new one grows the next year. Many of the delicate and most delicious species of bananas are too perishable to ship. Allergy to banana is quite common, especially in those sensitized to many fruits. The symptoms from such allergy may be extremely severe. Certain species of bananas are called plantain. This plantain in no way resembles the various species of English plantain, leaves of which are at times used as a salad in Europe and the pollen of which causes pollenosis in the spring.

Date (zizyphus lotus) grows on the date palm which is indigenous to Arabia and Egypt. Male and female trees exist. In cultivation, 1 male tree is grown for every 50 to 100 female ones and the flowers of the female tree are dusted with the pollen produced by the male. Many species of the date palm yield dates of different sizes and consistency. This nourishing fruit may be eaten raw or dried. It is made into a flour, an oil, and a wine in Arabia. Dates grown in southern California are gaining increasing favor in America.

Jujube (zizyphus jujuba) is a Chinese date brought from India over a thousand years ago. Another variety grows along the Mediterranean and also in California and Florida.

The Grape Family (Vitaceæ).—**Wild grapes** (vitis) grow throughout the world. By careful cultivation and selection, various edible varieties have been developed. The wine grape originated in Asia probably five thousand years ago and was later grown in Egypt, Europe, and America—nearly exclusively in California. The table grape was developed in America. The so-called northern fox grapes, native in this country, such as the

Concord, Catawba, Niagara, and Delaware, are used for grape juice and jellies. Some patients are allergic to one variety of grape and not to another. Grape seed oil in Europe is used as a salad oil.

Raisins are dried European or wine grapes. The dried *currant* used in cooking is a dried seedless raisin raised especially on the Grecian Islands of Zante.

Wines differ according to the variety of grape used. In dry wines, the grape sugar has all been fermented into alcohol; in sweet wines, the fermentation has been stopped by the addition of alcohol before the grape sugar has all been converted. Red wines are colored by the skin. White wines are made from white grapes or from colored grapes from which the skins have been removed. Yeast is used in the making of wines. **Brandy** is distilled from wine. **Cognac** is such a brandy made in that part of France. *Grape vinegar*, red or white, may be used by patients allergic to apple vinegar.

The Gooseberry Family (Grossulariaceæ).—Currant (ribes rubrum) was developed in northern Europe five or six hundred years ago. The red currant was brought from Europe to America. The Buffalo currant originated along the Missouri and Columbia Rivers and is cultivated at present in Utah. Several other varieties are raised. The berry is small with a tart flavor, used in jellies and preserves. Dried currants, as sold, are not real currants, but are dried small seedless raisins, especially from Grecian Islands.

Gooseberry (ribes grossularia) first grew in northern Europe. It was first cultivated in the 16th century. A native gooseberry also grew in New England. This berry is especially used in England where a large variety grows. They are used in jellies, jams, preserves, pies, and sauces.

The Rose Family (Rosaceæ).—These berries, used as foods, are related to roses and grow wild all over the world. During the last century, through cultivation, various species have been developed yielding larger and more delicious fruit.

Strawberry (fragaria) was so named because of its closeness to the ground as though it were strewed thereon. The berry is a carrier of seeds, which are on the surface of the fruit. Many patients suffer from urticaria due to this berry, and skin reactions often are absent. Lyon, as noted by Vaughan, observed strawberry allergy in four generations. (See page 55.)

Raspberry, Blackberry, Loganberry, Dewberry, Youngberry (rubus) are varieties of berries closely related. All are eaten fresh, or cooked into preserves, jellies, jams, frozen desserts, or in pies. The juices are used as flavors or in beverages.

The Huckleberry Family (Vacciniaceæ).—Vaughan states that members of this family grow from the tropics to the arctic areas, and include winter greens, teaberry, Labrador tea, rhododendron, azalea and trailing arbutus.   There are two important berries.

Huckleberry, blueberry, bilberry, indigenous to our country and eaten by the Indians, are used in preserves and pies.

Cranberry (vaccinium macrocarpon) is a native of North America.   The large type grows wild in bogs in the northern and eastern states and is cultivated in Wisconsin, Cape Cod and New Jersey especially.   The unopened flower resembles the head, bill, and neck of the crane.

Miscellaneous Fruits.—Tropical fruits and those of other countries gradually may be of value to the allergic patient, particularly if allergy exists to several of the commonly used fruits.

Guava (pisidium guajava) grows in tropical America.   The fruit looks like an orange and is used especially in a jelly.

Mango (curcuma amada) grows in most warm areas as in Mexico, Florida, and the West Indies.   It varies greatly in size, even up to that of a cantaloupe.   Fresh, canned, or preserved mango is eaten.

Avocado or alligator pear (persea gratissima) is native in tropical America and grows on a species of laurel.   It is now grown in all warm and tropical areas.   It is a member of the Laurel family to which cinnamon and bay leaves belong.

Papaya (papaw) (carica papaya) grows on a tree in tropical America.   It is usually eaten raw but may be boiled or preserved.

Persimmon (diospyros virginiana) is a plum-like fruit which is astringent until ripe.

Pomegranate (punica granatum) originated in tropical Asia and Africa.   It is a berry-like fruit, as large as an orange, with many seeds in a crimson edible pulp.

Vaughan calls attention to various fruits obtainable in Florida and New Orleans such as *mandarin, sapodilla, shaddock, chocho, monistera deliciosa, cherimoya or custard apple, carambola or star apple, prickly pear, kumquat, plantain, carissa, tamarind.*   He states that "The State of Florida, Department of Agriculture, Bulletin No. 46 (1935) gives a list of various tropical and subtropical fruits grown there.   The Agricultural Extension Service, Gainesville, Florida, Bulletin No. 85 (1936) contains many photographs and botanical descriptions of such fruits."

Nuts.—As already noted, the peanut (see page 82) and the almond (see page 88) are not nuts.   Allergy to nuts is quite frequent, especially to closely related ones as grouped below.

Walnut Family (Juglandeæ).—The English walnut originated in southwestern Asia and Asia Minor. Many varieties have been developed. A large percentage of the world's supply comes from the United States, especially California. The so-called black and white walnut or butternuts were indigenous in this country. Walnut oil made especially in Europe is used in cooking and on salads. Walnuts are frequent causes of canker sores and may produce other clinical manifestations. In California especially, the large black, and to a lesser extent, the English walnut trees pollinate profusely and severe nasal, bronchial and, at times, cutaneous allergies arise therefrom. Because of the frequency of such allergy to black walnut pollen, it is not wise to plant these trees for shade.

Pecan (carya olivæformis) was indigenous in Texas and the lower Mississippi Valley area. It is more closely related to hickory than to walnut.

Hickory (carya alba) is a native of this country.

Beech Family (Fagus).—Beech nuts (fagus ferruginea) are triangular, small and occur in pairs. In France, a coffee substitute is made from roasted nuts and in Germany a salad oil and butter substitute are made from the oil.

Chestnuts (castanea) originated in southern Europe and Asia. Vaughan states that chestnuts are an important food in certain districts in southern France, Italy, and Spain. The nuts are ground into flour, used in bread and desserts. One chestnut is indigenous to America along the eastern coast and the adjacent northern states. The chinquapin is a small variety growing in the southern states.

The *marron* is a large variety from France and Italy and is preserved or sugar coated. Roasted nuts of all varieties are favored.

The *horse chestnut* is bitter, though it has been used as a coffee substitute and in soups and gruels by Indians.

Filbert, Hazelnut, Cobnut (corylus) originated in Asia Minor and Europe and has been eaten since ancient times. The nuts are used as a source of oil in Russia. The hazelnut is indigenous in North America.

The following nuts are unrelated.

Brazil nuts or Niggertoes (bertholletia excelsa) come from a tropical tree of South America. The triangular nuts, usually 20 or so, fit into one large shell. This nut is not related to other foods.

Acorns (quercus esculus), used by the Indians, are still eaten in southern Europe.

Cashew nuts (anacardium occidentale) grew first in central and tropical South America and now in other tropical areas. They are not related to other nuts or common foods. Vaughan reported asthma and urticaria from this nut.

Cocoanuts (cocos nucifera) grow on a palm in the tropics of the Pacific and Indian Oceans. The meat may be eaten as such, grated and used in cakes, frostings, candies, and desserts. The milk is fairly palatable. The oil may be used in salad oils, oleo-margarines, in soaps and other commercial products.

Litchi nuts (litchi chinensis) come from the Chinese tree, now grown in the East Indies and India. The fruit has a hard covering, of soft white meat and a hard small dark seed. The dried fruit yields a black sweetish meat. One patient developed allergic headache and gastro-intestinal symptoms from this food. Canned fresh meat of the nut is available.

Pine nuts are eaten in many countries, especially the Himalayas, where the ground product is mixed with flour.

Fungi.—**Mushrooms**, as Vaughan states, are the fruit of a fungus growing up from the mycelium in the ground. Twelve or more varieties are edible. They are eaten as such and are used in sauces, soups, gravies, and other food mixtures. Severe allergy at times occurs to mushrooms.

Truffle grows in the ground without roots or upward shoots in Europe, especially France and also California. Its pleasant odor is recognized by trained dogs or hogs. It is used as a condiment in paté de foie gras and at times in sausage. Being sold in cans, it can be used in place of mushrooms when allergy to the latter exists.

Puffballs which are edible have a flavor similar to mushrooms but are not eaten much in this country.

Molds at times occur in cheeses (see page 70) and in certain fermented drinks in Japan.

Yeast is used in raised bakery and other food products, in fermented beverages, certain cheeses and, in recent years, very extensively as such, because of the vitamin content and heralded medicinal virtues. Allergy to yeast is rather common and skin testing with important varieties of yeasts should be routine. The regular pound cake or baker's yeast is pure with no added ingredients. The yeast cakes often contain a little tapioca and at times carotene in cottonseed oil because of its vitamin A content. When cottonseed allergy is present, its possible presence in yeast cakes should be remembered. Yeast allergy was also discussed on page 52.

Beverages.—**Coffee** (caffea arabica) was indigenous in Abyssinia from where it was taken to Arabia in the fifth century. This coffee was shipped from Mocha to Italy, Turkey, and later to

England.   Coffee houses were common.   The modern word "cafe" is thus explained.   Since the 17th century, coffee has been raised in Java, Central America, the Indies, and especially in Brazil. The roasting of the coffee bean releases a volatile oil, coffeol, which gives the aroma and flavor to coffee.   The bean becomes lighter and brown in color.   Allergy to coffee is not uncommon, being responsible for migraine, asthma, gastro-intestinal, cutaneous, and other manifestations in certain patients.

Allergy to adulterants of coffee, such as *chicory*, cereals, chestnuts, legumes, carrots and other substances may exist.   Many coffee substitutes also are made from various foods.   Vaughan lists a few, including dates, okra seeds, chicory, beech nuts, horse chestnuts, asparagus seeds, dried figs, and cereal grains.

Tea (camellia thea) originated in China where it has been a beverage for four or five thousand years.   Since the 17th century, its use spread to Europe and later to America.   A cup of tea contains about 1 to 2 grains of caffeine, about equal to that in a cup of coffee.   Whether allergy to one species of tea and not to others is present remains for future study.   Allergy to tea itself exists but less frequently than to coffee.

Chocolate (cocoa) (theobroma cacao) originated in Mexico, tropical South America and the Indies, and continues to grow in those areas.   The original Indian name was cocauntil.   The Spanish called it cocas and the English cocoa.   Spaniards first brought chocolate to Europe.   The height of the tree varies from 14 to 35 feet.   The pods containing the cocoa beans are 6 to 12 inches long.   Roasting enhances the flavor.   The final product is an oily dark, bitter fluid.   Sweet chocolate contains cocoa butter and sugar.   Condensed, powdered milk is added to milk chocolate.

Cocoa has less oil and cocoa butter than chocolate.

Cocoa butter is used in candies, ointments, cosmetics, and toilet preparations.

Allergy to **chocolate** is not infrequent.   Vaughan reports dermatitis from the local application of cocoa butter in a chocolate sensitive patient.

Maté (ilex paraguensis) is South American or Brazilian tea.   It grows on a species of holly.   Vaughan states that Brazil exports 120,000,000 pounds yearly.

The contents of beverages such as coca cola, root beer, beer, wines and whiskey are discussed on page 230.

Elderberry (sambucus nigra) is the fruit of a tree and is used to make elderberry wine and to color port wine in Portugal.   It is a member of the honeysuckle family and other edible foods are not related to it.

Spices and Condiments.—**Pepper** (black and white) (piper nigrum) grows on a climbing plant native in India, East Indies, and surrounding tropics. No closely allied plants yield food. It was used in Roman days. The unripe, dried, small berry makes black pepper. White pepper comes from the inside of the berry after the outer shell is removed. Pepper allergy is not unusual.

Peppers (capsicum) are discussed on page 84.

Vanilla (vanilla planifolia) comes from dried pods 6 to 10 inches long which grow on a climbing orchid vine native in Mexico. It is now grown in most tropical areas. The extract is an alcoholic extract of the bean. Imitation extracts are made with synthetic vanilla.

Nutmeg (myristica fragrans), indigenous in the East Indies, now grows in tropical countries and is the inner seed of a fruit which looks like a peach. **Mace** comes from the inner covering of the shell of nutmeg. The inside of the nut is the commercial nutmeg.

Allspice (pimenta officianalis) has a combined taste of several spices. It comes from the unripened dried seed of a tree growing in the East Indies.

Clove (engenia caryophyllata) comes from the tight bud of an evergreen tree indigenous in the Dutch Indies. It grows now in Africa and the East and West Indies. The oil of cloves is also used in cooking.

Cinnamon (cinnamomun cassia) is the inner bark of a tree of the laurel family which originated in Ceylon.

Bay leaves (laurus nobilis) are from another tree of the laurel family, native in the countries around the Mediterranean and in our southern states. They are not related to the bayberry from which bayrum is distilled.

Sage (salvia officinalis) leaves grow on a shrub, a member of the mint family. They are used in dressings of meats, fowl, to flavor sausages, meats, soups, cheese, and sauces.

Thyme (thymus vulgaris) leaves also grow on a shrub of the mint family and are used in dressings, sauces, and meats.

Mint (mentha), including peppermint, spearmint, and penny royal, are used as flavors, the oil being extracted from the leaves. Mint leaves are also used to season meats.

Peppermint (mentha piperita) oil comes from the dark green leaves and flowers of the aromatic mint. Essence of peppermint is a solution of this oil in alcohol.

Spearmint (mentha spicata) is the common garden mint used as a flavor which depends on its aromatic oil.

Savory (micromeria juliana) is an herb indigenous in the countries around the Mediterranean. It belongs to the mint family. The leaves are used for seasoning.

Wintergreen (gaultheria procumbens) is a North American herb whose leaves yield the aromatic oil. It consists mostly of methyl salicylate. Thus, the synthetic salicylate or birch oil is usually sold as oil of wintergreen or gaultheria oil. Birch belongs to the Beech family discussed on page 92.

Tarragon (artemesis dracuncillus) is an aromatic sage used for seasoning. It flavors a brand of vinegar.

Marjoram is a fragrant herb used in cooking.

Poppy seeds are used in baking and as condiments. The oil is used in salads, iodized oil and in industry.

Mustard and horse-radish have been discussed on page 81.

Licorice (hedysarum mackenzii) comes from the dried root of a plant native in Russia and Central Asia, which is related to the legumes. It is used in candy, tobacco, in certain liqueurs and porter and to flavor foods.

Fennel, caraway seeds, aniseed and dill have been described on page 83.

Ginger (zingiber officinale) is the root or root stock of a plant which grows tall leaves each year. It grows in moist, tropical regions in the West Indies, Africa, and the East Indies. It is used in ginger ale, candies, and spiced meats and sauces. Jamaica ginger is its alcoholic extract. The ingredients of ginger ale are listed on page 230.

Oils.—**Cottonseed oil** (gossypium) is pressed from the seeds of cotton. It is used in salad dressings and mayonnaise. It may be an adulterant of olive and other oils. Hydrogenated, it forms a solid fat, sold as Crisco, mixed with lard in Snowdrift, or used with other fats to make oleomargarine. It is added to canned fish of various types and is used in certain soaps.

Sensitization to cottonseed allergen, especially by inhalation, may be as severe as any encountered. (See page 47.) Such patients usually cannot take any cottonseed oil or fat by mouth without severe symptoms. Nuts, blanched or treated with such oil, may cause allergy. Vaughan notes the variation in the various fats and oils used in commercial salad oils and shortenings. He found 189 brands containing cottonseed oils with other fats.

Olive oil is pressed from olives (see Olive) grown especially in California, France, and Italy. Virgin oil comes from the first pressing. The second pressing yields so-called "foots," used in soaps and as a commercial oil. Much imported olive oil is adulterated with cottonseed, tea seed, corn, peanut, or sesame oils. Prepared mayonnaise may contain any of these oils.

Sesame oil is pressed from the seeds of an East Indian herb (sesamum indicum). The seeds are also used as a food and in cooking.

Peanut oil, corn oil, cocoanut oil and walnut oil, have been discussed previously.

MISCELLANEOUS FOODS

Olives (olea europæa) grow on trees indigenous in the Mediterrean area. They are common in California and yield profusely. Green and ripe olives are pickled with brine and vinegar, and various condiments such as fennel, laurel leaves, thyme, coriander, or various peppers may be added. Allergy to olive pollen may produce severe nasobronchial or cutaneous manifestations. Such patients may be allergic to the olives and their oil. One patient had severe abdominal cramping and gas from olive oil allergy.

Privet, grown in gardens, is closely related to olive.

Hop (humulus lupulus) gives a bitter taste to beer, being used for this reason even in ancient Rome. Allergy to the pollen is not uncommon.

Marshmallow (althæa officinalis) is related to cotton and originated in the sea marshes of Europe and Asia. The roots yield a colorless gum used in mucilage and, at times, in medicines. Formerly the candy marshmallow was made of this. Its present content is noted on page 245.

Sapodilla (Achras sapota) or **Chicle** is a solidified sap or latex of the Acheas tree which is indigenous in Central and South America. Gum is made of chicle to which flavors, sugar or corn syrup are added. Allergy to chicle has been reported causing severe nasal blocking, sneezing, itching, with asthma.

Bamboo shoots are eaten by Chinese and Japanese and are being introduced into American cooking in certain areas. Canned shoots are available.

Sugars. — Cane sugar is described on page 64. Corn sugar is described on page 64. Beet sugar is described on page 79. Sorghum molasess is described on page 64.

Maple sugar comes from several varieties of the maple tree (aceraceæ saccharinum). The rock or sugar maple indigenous in New England yields much sugar. Most commercial syrups contain cane or corn sugars. Some pure maple sugars and syrups are on the market.

7

Karaya gum (sterculi aceæ) comes from the bark of a tree of the Astragalus species. At times, it is called Indian tragacanth or sterculia gum and belongs to the group of bassorim gums. This and other gums and vegetable mucilages in the dry state absorb large amounts of water—several times as much even as agar. Figley states that karaya gum contains 0.1 per cent total nitrogen. Inhalation allergy to karaya gum is discussed on page 46.

Karaya gum, according to Bullen and Figley, is included in gum drops and jelly beans and other soft center fillers, in ice cream, ices, and ice cream powders, certain diabetic and health foods, certain brands of junket and gelatin, fillers in various pies, flavor emulsions, and some salad dressings. It is also used in various hand lotions, and especially in wave-setting solutions, as discussed on page 46, in tooth pastes such as Listerine and Lactana, in denture adhesive powders such as Dr. Wernet's powder, Dent-a-Firm, Denture powder and Stix, and many laxatives such as Karaba, Karabim, Saraka, Mucara, Imbicoll, and Bassoran. It is used in the wrappers of certain cigars.

Agar-agar is an algæ or Japanese seaweed. It is used in laxatives to increase the bulk in the intestinal canal, and also to thicken jellies, ice cream, and in diabetic foods. Vaughan found an iodine allergy produced by iodine in agar agar.

Irish Moss (carragheen or pearl moss) is an edible seaweed gathered on the shores of the British Isles and northern states of our country. It is used in blanc mange and, at times, in jellies.

Gum acacia or gum arabic (see page 46) comes from several species of acacia trees and is composed chiefly of calcium, magnesium, and potassium salts of arabic acid. It is used in adhesives, inks, confections, especially lozenges, and medical emulsions, and may be injected intravenously.

Psyllium seeds, used so frequently for cathartic purposes, may produce allergy and cause various allergic manifestations.

Honey produces severe allergy due to bee allergen. Pollen in the honey may also cause specific symptoms.

DYES, DRUGS AND CHEMICALS

Dyes, used to color foods, candies, gelatins and drinks, may produce various manifestations of allergy. Thus, Baer reported dermatitis of the skin and cramping in the abdomen from a green dye in ingested gelatin. (See page 26.) *Phenolphthalein* is responsible for the pink color in most foods, candies, and gums, dentrifices and medicines, and is used in many cathartics. It is responsible for many types of skin and mucous membrane lesions.

Drugs taken by mouth are especially productive of allergic dermatoses which may continue for weeks or even years after their discontinuance. *Barbiturates, bromides, iodides, arsenic compounds, quinine, phenolphthalein, acetanilide-antipyrin* compounds and any other drug may be causative. *Acetylsalicylic acid* (aspirin), especially, may produce urticaria and angioneurotic edema, severe and even fatal asthma, and gastro-intestinal symptoms in sensitized patients. The doctor, therefore, must carefully obtain a drug history as discussed on page 21.

Iodine allergy most frequently produces nasal congestion, headache, swelling of the submaxillary and sublingual glands. Fever may result, and acne-like pimples, especially after a week or two of iodine or iodide therapy are common. More extensive dermatitis may occur in markedly sensitive patients—those in whom such a rash develops after the application of iodine to a small cut.

Agranulocytosis, characterized by disappearance of the granular white cells in the blood and necroses in the gums, often leading to to death, is probably due to allergy in the blood forming bone-marrow cells, especially from amidopyrine, a drug used for headaches or pain. Other drugs such as arsphenamine, sulfanilamide, gold salts, and dinitrophenol also may be responsible.

Mineral and organic substances in drinking water may produce allergic manifestations in the gastro-intestinal tract, skin, or other body tissues. *Chlorine* in water may produce dermatitis. Pollen in water probably causes symptoms in certain sensitized patients. Products of vegetable growths, or animal life in the water itself or in the soil or on walls of reservoirs, tanks, pipes, or viaducts holding drinking water may cause sensitization in rare individuals.

CONTACTANTS

Contact dermatitis or eczema is due to sensitization in the superficial epidermal cells of the skin and may arise to practically any substance which contacts the skin, even to the infinitesimal amounts of the volatile resin from poison ivy and other vegetations which may be in the air. Whether the active allergenic substance has to combine with a protein of the skin to which allergy then develops or whether the active allergen itself creates the epidermal sensitization is not known. *Sensitization in the skin of a monkey to a chemical substance experimentally produced seems to spread from the original site throughout the rest of the body's skin.* Such spread of allergy is evidenced by the following: If the original site is on the foreleg and a cuff of the skin is cut out above this site, the rest of the skin of the animal does not become sensitized.   Sensitization to these contact allergens, moreover, seems to vary in degree in different areas of the skin.   This contact eczema is often called *dermatitis venenata.*

Contact dermatitis may develop rapidly after a single slight or brief repeated exposures to the allergenic substance.   This seems to be true of poison ivy and oak, since most people living in an area where they grow become allergic thereto.   At times such contact allergy only develops after prolonged and marked contact with the substance and especially if absence from contact in such an individual persists for three or more weeks during which contact allergy develops.   When people are working with substances, such as rubber, lacquers, or other chemicals, therefore, which are apt to cause contact allergy, complete freedom from contact with such substances during vacations or lay-offs might not be advisable.

Contact allergy is studied by so-called patch tests.   The suspected substance, overlaid with a small piece of cellophane, is applied to the skin by a strip of adhesive tape for approximately forty-eight hours.   The degree of reaction varies from a slight erythema to marked vesiculation and oozing.   When severe allergy is present, the burning and itching may develop in one or two hours, necessitating removal of the testing material.   If mild allergy is present, the roughness, redness, and scaling of the skin may not develop for two to five days, showing the necessity of observing the test areas for several days after the initial forty-eight hours.   Test substances which are volatile, such as the ether or acetone extracts of the resins of leaves of plants, may be applied to a small skin area without subsequent covering with adhesive, as advised by Shelmire.   Reactions to the substance may vary in different skin areas, often being most marked near the area in which eczema is present.   Positive reactions may only occur, moreover, in the presence of heat, friction, or other influences present when the dermatitis originally developed.

Differentiation is necessary between substances which are skin irritants and which produce allergy.   Those which produce a reaction in every skin, such as certain acids, alkalis, and turpentine, are irritants.   Certain substances in strong concentrations are irritants but may also produce allergy.   Thus, a dilution which fails to react on the normal skin must be used for patch testing.

To list the tremendous number of substances to which contact allergy may arise is prohibitive.   Tests must be made with those suspected by the patient or by the physician through a careful analysis of the history and his various contacts at home, work or recreation.   Each home, trade, profession, occupation, or recreation entails contact with materials such as chemicals, dyes, soaps, dentifrices, perfumes, cosmetics, plants, flowers, bulbs, fabrics, furnishings, clothing, lacquer, varnishes, paints, turpentine, woods, furniture polishes, waxes, oils, gasoline, glue, cement, rubber, vulcanizers, foods, spices, yeasts, metals, metal polishes, celluloid, bakelite, formalin, insecticides (including pyrethrum), antiseptics, anesthetics, drugs, and medicaments. The variety of contacts possible in recreation are obvious in horsemen, boatsmen, golfers, hunters, painters, gardeners, wood workers, photographers, musicians, and animal lovers; and in each industrial occupation, many special substances, organic and inorganic, demand consideration.

Cosmetics and toilet articles used by the patient, relatives, or, at times, by friends, are especially prone to develop contact eczema.   Some of these follow: hair tonics, scalp lotions, hair, eyebrow, and eyelash dyes, eyebrow pencils, creams of all types, cleaning lotions, astringents, face, body, and dusting powders, rouges, lipsticks, nail paints, nail polishes, cuticle removers, and other manicuring aids, perfumes, mascara, freckle removers, hair removers, eyelash curlers, combs, hair ornaments, sunburn lotions, nasal drops and sprays, eye drops, deodorants, contraceptives, douching powders, menstrual pads, mouth washes, dentures, dentifrices, dental floss, hair setting solutions, and substances such as egg or orris root in wet or dry shampoos.   Any one of the many chemical or organic ingredients in any of the above preparations may produce contact allergy.   Patch testing with such ingredients often reveals the offenders.

Clothing and wearing apparel may produce dermatitis.   Wool, silk, mohair, cotton, rayon, or linen, either plain or dyed, may be responsible.   Dyed stockings, underwear, or night clothes which contact the skin should be laundered before wearing, especially if susceptibility to contact allergy is suspected.   Certain chemicals used to "finish" fabrics are productive of contact allergy.

Dyes of various types may cause dermatitis.   Simon and Rackemann reported dermatitis to a blue dye which necessitated patch tests with a small amount of the fabric of every suit, hat, tie, sock, or other dyed material worn to determine its possible allergic reactivity.   Dyes in shoes may produce local or even generalized dermatitis.

Allergy to rubber or various ingredients in rubber materials, as in girdles, garters, stockings or dentures, may occur.   *Phosphorus* allergy is responsible for so-called match-box dermatitis from matches carried in a pocket.   *Nickel* dermatitis may arise under spectacle rims, garter buckles, or wrist watches.   Allergy to *tortoise shell rims* of glasses has been noted.   Further possibilities of these types, of course, are obvious.

Oils and resins of vegetations are very important.   *Poison oak and ivy* are most common causes of contact dermatitis.   *Primrose* and many other flowering plants, such as *daffodils, narcissus, jonquils, sage, pyrethrum, chrysanthemum, pansy, bleeding heart, gaillardia, and verbena* are reported causes of contact dermatitis. Trees and weeds, such as *acacia, elm, helenium, cocklebur, ragweed, camomile, marsh elder*, have been found to cause contact dermatitis. The resins and oils in the skins of fruits such as citrus fruits, of vegetables, meats, and other food products may cause dermatitis on the hands and other skin areas of housewives, cooks, food handlers, and food cultivators.

Further comment is of interest concerning *drugs and medicaments* which cause contact allergy.   Ephedrine in nose drops, belladonna in eye drops, hexylresorcinol in tooth paste, or for local skin application, iodine or benzoin on the skin, novocaine, nupercaine, or other anesthetics on the skin or mucous membranes, quinine and chloral in hair lotions and tonics, mercury, arsenic, balsam of Peru, butysin picrate, and many other chemicals, drugs, and essential oils in lotions, salves, or ointments locally applied cause contact dermatitis of the skin, scalp, or mucous membranes. Egg or orris shampoos produce urticaria or dermatitis in the scalp of sensitized people.

Sensitization to various ingredients in *soaps* must be remembered.   Some skins are susceptible to the natural irritants in soaps. Patch tests with various soaps used, therefore, must be interpreted with these facts in mind.

Contact dermatitis in industry and the manifold occupations has received much study in the last thirty or more years and its many causes and ramifications have been discussed in a recent book by Schwartz and Tulipan.   It is recognized that certain workers are more prone to develop this type of allergy and have skins more susceptible to skin irritants than others.   Tests to discover such susceptible workers are recommended and a type of work can thus be chosen for them which is not associated with great danger of contact sensitizations.   An additional discussion of contact dermatitis is on page 121.

INFECTANT AND DISEASED TISSUE SENSITIZATION

Koch in 1882, in his epochal studies on tuberculosis, described a red papular reaction to tuberculin injected into the skin which appeared in twenty-four to forty-eight hours.   *This delayed type of reaction was responsible for the word "allergy" which Von Pirquet suggested for this altered tissue reactivity.* Such delayed reactions also are known to develop in smallpox, diphtheria, typhoid, pneumonia, and other infections. They indicate the presence of allergy to the products of the causative bacteria or viruses. Such reactions, moreover, arise to various yeasts and fungi, causing diseased processes in man. Their importance in diagnosis is obvious.

The immediate wheal type of skin reaction, described on page 23, usually present in pollen or food allergy, rarely occurs in bacterial allergy. This may be due to the continued presence of infection in the patient. Of *interest is the probability that this delayed tissue reaction produces more tissue destruction than does the immediate wheal type of reaction.* Such delayed and continued allergic reactions to infectant products probably lead to many of the tissue changes arising from infection. The protective nature of allergy arising from such infectant allergens, however, is of great importance. As allergy and immunity develop, acute infections, such as measles, chicken pox, scarlet fever, gradually are overcome. Without tuberculin allergy with the walling off of inspired or harbored tubercular bacilli, the disease would spread, and arrest of the infection would be impossible.

As stated above, *yeasts and fungi* which produce disease in the skin and, less often, in other body tissues result in allergy. In patients affected with epidermophytosis or athlete's foot, sensitization to the allergen of the causative fungus may result in an eruption on the hands or other skin areas. *Such lesions are called epidermophytids.* They arise from blood-borne allergens or spores from the feet or other actively infected tissue. Other "id" eruptions to bacterial allergens probably occur due to foci of infection in a tissue distant from the actual skin lesions.

Bacterial allergy may arise to the streptococci, staphylococci, or other bacteria in foci of infection in teeth, tonsils, sinuses, prostate, gall-bladder, appendix, pelvic, rectal, or other tissues of the body. Such allergy probably affects every cell of the body, and if exaggerated in any special area, symptoms such as asthma, hay fever, arthritis or urticaria may develop. Bacterial allergy as a major cause of such manifestations, especially of bronchial asthma and hay fever, is much less frequent than was assumed fifteen or twenty years ago. The probable rôle of bacterial allergy in the production of clinical symptoms will be discussed in Chapter IV.

Allergy to parasites in the body tissues may produce tissue disturbances in the affected tissues or in distant areas. Intestinal parasites, especially round worms, have been responsible for asthma. Allergy to other parasites likewise is possible. Echinococcus in the liver or lungs results in a high degree of allergy which may produce severe allergic shock with asthma, urticaria and other allergic symptoms when the infected tissues are incised with the release of the allergen into the blood stream.

Allergy to the products of diseased or injured tissues may occur. A severe reaction in the eye may arise after a second cataract operation, due to the sensitization arising to the lens protein absorbed during the previous cataract operation. (See page 136.) In the same way, allergy may develop to the products of diseased or infected tissues in the body, though unquestioned proof of such allergy is not easy to obtain.

INSECT BITES

The *papules, swelling, erythema, and itching resulting from the bites of mosquitoes, fleas, bed bugs, lice, ticks, flies, bees,* or *similar insects are the results of allergy established by previous bites by the same type of insect.* At times, hives in distant skin areas, asthma, hay fever, and even gastro-intestinal symptoms may arise when the allergy is exaggerated. Severe urticaria, nausea, asthma, falling blood-pressure, shock and even death have been known to result from allergy to bee and wasp venom.

Hyposensitization with extracts of the insect in question reduces the patient's susceptibility to the bite. This has been done with antigens of mosquitoes, lake flies, bees, wasps, and fleas.

INJECTANTS

As outlined on page 36, *allergy may result from sera, drugs, vaccines, vitamins, hormones, and other ingredients in ductless gland products and their chemical substitutes, administered to the patient.* The allergens themselves given to pollen, animal emanation, dust, or other types of sensitive patients can always produce or exaggerate allergic symptoms if given in too large doses. These various injectants are most frequently administered subcutaneously or intradermally. Sera, drugs, vaccines, vitamins, or allergens are often given intravenously; drugs and foods are given by rectum; and drugs, sera, and, at times, allergens are introduced into the nasal, sinal, aural cavities, into the urogenital, vaginal, bronchial or cerebrospinal spaces for diagnostic or therapeutic reasons. The possibility of localized, distant, or generalized allergic reactions from any one of these substances must be remembered. Such allergy is more likely in patients who have a definite allergic tendency, particularly to the development of drug allergies.

Allergy to serum proteins, injected for the prevention and especially the treatment of diphtheria, tetanus, pneumonia, cerebrospinal meningitis, and other infections, is important to remember. A rare individual—about 1 in 50,000 to 70,000—is naturally so allergic to horse serum proteins that the injection of an extremely small dose produces an allergic reaction which may be rapidly fatal. Many others are sensitive to a lesser degree, especially if serum has been given previously. Within a few minutes, hours, or in a few days after its administration, they develop allergic symptoms of so-called serum sickness, characterized by redness, swelling, and hives of the skin, at times of the entire body, wheezing or asthma, congestion and suffusion of the conjunctivæ and nasal membranes, fever, joint pains and swellings, headache, and other less common symptoms. Symptoms occurring in a few hours to six or seven days are usually due to previous sensitization arising from former serum therapy and at times from allergy to the inhaled emanations or ingested meat of the horse or other animal whose serum is being given. (See page 73.) Serum sickness, developing in from seven to fourteen days, is due in nearly every case to the interaction of the serum proteins still present in the patient's blood and tissues with the reacting bodies of allergy developed to the recently injected serum proteins. Any severe symptoms require the hypodermic administration of epinephrine 1 to 1000 as necessary for relief, and the local and general therapy advised by the physician. Recently, histaminase, a ferment which breaks down histamine given by mouth has proved of benefit in some of these patients with serum sickness.

Before serum is administered, the physician must make preliminary tests to determine any possible serum allergy. Such tests and serum administration are discussed on page 226.

Other drugs, vaccines, hormones, and vitamins must also be given with the possibility of allergy in mind. This is especially true when the patient gives a history of any idiosyncrasy or intolerance to medicines or drugs taken in former years. It is often wise to give a small initial dose of any of these to ascertain any possible allergy that may exist before the regular doses are taken.

Iodine allergy, especially, is quite common. Thus, before iodized oil is injected intrabronchially or in any other cavity of the body or before an iodine containing drug is given by vein, any possible allergy should be determined by giving iodides or the drug in question by mouth for a day or two.   Patients must be informed about possible allergy to iodides as presented on page 114.

Arsenic containing drugs, such as the arsphenamines and cacodylates, are given subcutaneously or intravenously.   Allergy to such drugs may develop at any time during the patient's treatment and if further arsenical drugs are given by mouth or injection in the slightest amount, skin rashes, associated with itching and even severe generalized scaling dermatitis, may develop which is very persistent and at times endangers life.   Such arsenic allergy continues until all of the drug has been thrown off from the body. If the slightest amount continues to enter the body, as from the eating of arsenic sprayed fruit or vegetables or from mineral waters or impure medicines or from the inhalation of dust of houses in which traces of arsenic from wall paper or fumigated carpets or fabrics are present, then the dermatitis will persist.

Drugs for nervousness, sleep or anesthesia may be given hypodermically, intravenously, or by rectum as well as by mouth. Various *barbital* derivatives, *cocaine, procaine*, and other similar drugs may produce allergy, especially in patients with a personal or family history of other drug idiosyncrasies.   If itching or skin rashes or other unusual symptoms develop while these or other drugs are being taken, the drugs should be discontinued until the physician is consulted.

Allergy to *iron* or its compounds at times occurs.   Gastrointestinal symptoms are particularly frequent.   Its injection or oral administration produces symptoms in sensitized patients.

Evidence is accumulating that *allergy may develop to the pure chemical vitamins* such as to *thiamin* (vitamin B) and *cevitamic acid* (vitamin C) when given by mouth, subcutaneously, or intravenously.   *Milk sensitive patients* develop various allergic manifestations when milk or its proteins are given intramuscularly for so-called non-specific protein therapy, or when given with barium in enemas for colon x-ray studies.   *Allergens of milk and other foods may be present in the blood of a donor* and cause allergic symptoms in a patient specifically sensitive to such foods.   Thus donors usually are asked to fast for three to four hours before being used for a transfusion.

The probability that allergy develops to *catgut, silk or other sutures and ligatures* used in surgery, buried as they are in the body tissues, has led to the use of material least likely to produce sensitization.   Such suture allergy may prevent wound healing and lead to inflammation.   A fine, rustless, steel thread has been adopted by certain surgeons.

Ingredients in *douches, contraceptives, and vaginal medicaments* may produce allergy. One patient had asthma and nasal allergy from the rose perfume in a contraceptive.

PLACENTAL AND MOTHER'S MILK TRANSMITTED ALLERGENS

Food allergens ingested by the mother may pass through the placenta into the blood of the fetus and produce sensitization. Sensitization of the fetus to drugs, inhalants, and bacteria also is possible but difficult to prove. Babies are rarely born with actual allergic manifestations, though allergic dermatitis is at times present at birth. Such intrauterine sensitization probably accounts for the allergic symptoms which at times arise to the first foods given.

Mother's milk contains infinitesimal amounts of food allergens from the mother's diet, sufficient to produce allergic symptoms in markedly sensitive infants. With the exclusion of such foods from the mother's diet, the baby's allergy, at times, will disappear.

PHYSICAL ALLERGY

Various symptoms of allergy may develop in certain individuals when exposed to *cold, heat, and sunlight.* Duke, especially, has studied these reactions. It is probable that these physical agents change the proteins of the body tissues with an abnormal release of histamine or a similar substance or that sensitization is established to such changed proteins. Urticaria from heat or cold, dermatitis from sunlight, and certain nasal and bronchial symptoms such as wheezing and nasal congestion and swelling, together with generalized symptoms, most frequently arise from such physical allergy. They may be associated with ingestant or inhalant sensitizations. Moreover, cold, heat, and other physical agents may release or activate an underlying food or inhalant allergy which otherwise would produce no symptoms. Such factors may, therefore, be secondary in their action and are discussed below.

SECONDARY FACTORS

It has long been recognized that bronchial asthma in particular and also hay fever or nasal allergy, allergic headache, and various dermatoses, especially atopic dermatitis, are exaggerated by so-called non-specific causes. *Dusts of all types*, especially in inhalant sensitive patients, may exaggerate symptoms even when allergy does not exist to them. *Soap powders* are irritant even to normal people. *Odors, smokes, and chemical fumes*, especially of sulphur, formaldehyde, and paint produce such effects. *Changes in temperature, weather, humidity*, and wind may precipitate symptoms. The effect of seasons and of proximity to the ocean, especially on food allergy, was discussed on page 58. The *allergic balance may be upset by various acute and chronic infections*, especially by head or bronchial colds. However, *the frequent mistake of attributing the nasal manifestations of perennial hay fever or those nasal symptoms which often precede an asthmatic attack to an infectious cold must not be made.* (See page 110.) It appears that the increase or onset of bronchial asthma, urticaria, or migraine, or sick headache during *menstruation* is due to the heightening of the tissue reactivity occurring before or during the period. The failure of glandular therapy to relieve these manifestations confirms this opinion. The disappearance of various symptoms of allergy during pregnancy is explained by the state of *anergy* (inability to react to allergenic causes) which develops in many pregnant women. *Indigestion, overeating, and constipation may lower the threshold of reaction* so that allergic symptoms are increased or arise. Finally, *neurosis, nervousness, and excitement secondarily activate potential* or *active allergies in many patients.*

At times, *the symptoms themselves are wrongly attributed to these secondary, non-specific causes, largely because the physician cannot discover the allergens which are responsible.* In such cases, continued study and treatment of the patient from the allergic viewpoint is obviously important.

CHAPTER IV

CLINICAL ALLERGY AND ITS CONTROL

BECAUSE of the limited scope of this handbook, the discussion of the manifestations of allergy and their therapeutic control must be brief. The types of allergy usually responsible for such symptoms, the indications for the use of elimination diets, the procedures necessary for the control of inhalant, bacterial, and contact allergy, will be outlined. Other types of therapy, useful in the alleviation of the various symptoms will be mentioned. For a more complete discussion of the writer's experience in the diagnosis and treatment of all these manifestations with a discussion of the literature, the reader is referred to the writer's text entitled "Clinical Allergy" (1937). Other textbooks by Vaughan, Tuft, Rackemann, Coca, Walzer and Thommen, Fineberg, and Balyeat, contain valuable theoretical and practical information.

Before discussing the various clinical manifestations of allergy, *it is necessary to stress the great importance of a complete physical examination, laboratory, and x-ray studies, so that all existent pathology is discovered and all possible causes, other than allergy, of the symptomatology are considered.*

BRONCHIAL ASTHMA AND ALLERGIC BRONCHITIS

The diagnosis of bronchial asthma must be made by the physician with a realization that all dyspnea, wheezing, and coughing are not due to this disease. Obstructions, growths, and inflammations in the throat, larynx, and bronchi, foreign bodies in the bronchial tract, goiters, tumors around the trachea or in the mediastinum, decompensation of the heart, aneurysms, pneumonia, pulmonary tuberculosis and other pulmonary inflammations, pulmonary tumors, atelectasis, fluid in the chest cavity, the alkalosis resulting from hyperventilation due to nervousness, and neuroses themselves may yield symptoms which have been mistaken for bronchial asthma. On the other hand, patients with bronchial asthma have been treated for pneumonia, heart disease, emphysema, and other conditions. These considerations, of course, emphasize the necessity of an accurate diagnosis of bronchial asthma by means of a skillfully taken history, careful physical examination, and necessary x-ray and laboratory studies, discussed in Chapter II.

(109)

Recurrent or chronic bronchitis is often due to the same causes responsible for bronchial asthma. Wheezing and difficult breathing are absent, due to a minimum of mucosal swelling, production of mucus and smooth muscle spasm in the bronchi. All causes of bronchitis due to infection, especially tuberculosis, must be ruled out by physical examination, x-ray, and laboratory tests conducted by the physician.

Bronchial asthma, due to food allergy, tends to recur throughout the year, especially from the early fall to late spring, being most severe in January and February in North America. *The beneficial effect of the summer months and of dry inland areas discussed on page* 58 must be realized. In children and often in adults, bronchial asthma due to food allergy usually occurs in attacks, often preceded by a so-called head cold due to the allergy first affecting the nasal and sinusal tissues for one or two days before the pulmonary tissues are markedly affected. Such attacks may recur every few days or weeks according to the degree of food allergy which exists. After an attack, lasting for one to five or more days, at times associated with allergic fever or actual secondary pulmonary infection, nausea, vomiting, and prostration, a refractory period may develop lasting for a few days or weeks. The "reacting bodies" in the pulmonary tissues have been exhausted during the explosive asthmatic attacks and the causative foods can thus be eaten for days or weeks without asthma until such "reacting bodies" again accumulate sufficiently so that their union with the food allergens again produces the nasal and later the bronchial manifestations. As such recurrent asthma continues, often absent or reduced during the summer, the attacks may become less severe, more persistent and finally a chronic type of bronchial asthma results which may be exaggerated at intervals. In older patients, *food allergy may be responsible for such perennial asthma of years' duration.* Superimposed may be a low grade infectious bronchitis and when large amounts of purulent sputum are expectorated, the physician must study the possibility of complicating bronchiectasis with iodized oil instillations and the x-ray. Precautions in the use of iodized oil were noted on page 114. As previously emphasized, *food allergy often is complicated with inhalant allergy of varying types and bacterial allergy occasionally may be a marked or minor cause.*

Ingestant allergy due to various drugs may cause bronchial asthma. Aspirin or acetylsalicylic acid seems to exaggerate or cause such symptoms in about 20 per cent of all patients with bronchial asthma. Other ingested drugs rarely cause bronchial allergy.

Inhalant allergy is also a most important cause of bronchial asthma. Moreover, it is often associated with food allergy in the etiology. When *pollen allergy* is operative, the symptoms occur in the spring, summer, or fall months according to the causative pollens, and nasal allergy or hay fever is usually present. Bronchial asthma due to severe pollen allergy may persist with moderate amelioration through the winter months, possibly due to pollen in house dust, but usually due to food or, rarely, to bacterial allergy. *Air-borne spores of fungi* occasionally cause other inhalant allergies as noted on page 51. Bronchial asthma due to *animal emanations* always needs consideration, especially when the history of animal contacts is obtained and when positive skin reactions are present. The many sources of animal emanations in pillows, mattresses, furniture, carpets, pads under carpets and rugs, on friends' and relatives' clothing, and from other sources are discussed in Chapter III. *Dusts*, encountered in working, recreational and, especially, in home environments, are common causes of inhalation bronchial asthma. Skin reactions are frequently positive, especially when extracts of the actual dusts encountered by the patient are made. Bronchial asthma, moreover, often arises to the so-called *miscellaneous inhalants*, including kapok and cottonseed allergens, especially from old mattresses, pillows, and furniture, from orris root, karaya gum, pyrethrum, silk, flaxseed, and glue dust—all of which may be inhaled as such or which may be in house or in other types of dusts. All of these inhalants have been individually discussed in Chapter III.

Bacterial allergy as a cause of bronchial asthma or allergic bronchitis is rare but, as noted on page 102, when it is present, its recognition and control are mandatory.

Finally, *neurogenic asthma* is necessary to keep in mind. Such may also arise in patients affected with ingestant or inhalant asthma, particularly in nervously unstable and anxious individuals.

The *diagnosis of the various ingestant and inhalant causes of bronchial allergy* has been discussed in Chapter III. It was noted therein that, *when food allergy is suspected, trial diet should be used for several weeks for diagnostic study.* For this, the Cereal-free Elimination Diets 1, 2, and 3, menus for which are given on page 157 for adults, and on page 184 for children, have been of most value. The occasional patient in whom test negative diets can be used is discussed on page 14. *The failure to use elimination diets properly and over a sufficient period of time accounts, in the writer's opinion, for the inability to relieve a great number of patients in this country today with chronic bronchial asthma who have food allergy as the sole or an important secondary cause of their symptoms.* When legume allergy is suspected, then Diets 1 and 2 as given on page 161 may be used, and other elimination and supplemental diets may be necessary before the possibilities of food allergy can finally be determined.

The *time necessary for adequate diet trial,* as noted on page 141, must be remembered. With all such diet trial, moreover, *proper nutrition and weight maintenance must be assured.* This is possible when the elimination diets and their menus are used as detailed Chapter V. The final determination of specific food allergies by gradual additions of individual foods to the diet when the patient has been symptom-free for a period longer than was usual before diet trial, can be made according to the suggestions on the use of diet trial on pages 145 and 155.

When chronic bronchial asthma is present, inhalant allergy as well as food allergy should be suspected until relief occurs. Then the rôle of one or both of these types of allergy can be determined as the patient continues his coöperation with the physician. As discussed on page 25, skin reactions to allergenic inhalants may be negative or indefinite, but this occurs less often than to allergenic foods. If inhalant allergy is probable, the *establishment of environmental control* in the patient's bedroom and in his living and working environments is most important. If the symptoms are serious or if a partial environmental control has not produced relief, then the strict control as discussed on page 31 should be established. This is especially necessary in the intractable type of asthma and may best be accomplished in a proper hospital room. *With such control, and with the accurately prepared elimination diet noted above, together with the hyposensitization therapy next discussed and the medical procedures suggested below, there are only a few cases of severe or intractable bronchial asthma that do not respond and in which the causative allergens cannot be gradually determined.*

When pollen allergy is indicated by history, skin testing or the results of environmental control, then hyposensitization with proper antigens and technic as discussed in Chapter III must be done often over a period of months or years. Relief, however, is usually possible in a few days with co-seasonal therapy. (See page 41.) *When animal emanation and miscellaneous inhalant allergies are indicated by history, skin testing, or the results of environmental control, hyposensitization with proper antigens is also usually necessary.* If the sources of such inhalants can be eliminated from the patient's environment, such therapy may not be required. As noted on page 39, the antigens must contain active allergens of the specific allergenic substances affecting the patient. Doses must be given and increased conservatively and symptoms must never be reproduced or exaggerated by such injections. *House dust allergy* necessitates proper environmental control. Hyposensitization is very beneficial in most of these patients but should be done with properly prepared autogenous dust extracts. (See page 48.) The same applies when allergy exists to other occupational and environmental dusts such as to feed and grain dusts in the dairy, livestock or chicken businesses.

The *medicinal treatment of the symptoms of bronchial asthma* requires brief comment in this handbook. For the relief of symptoms, the *hypodermic administration of 1 to 1000 epinephrine solution* in from 0.1 to 0.8 cc. according to the age of the patient and the severity of the asthma is of greatest value. Small doses repeated every two to five minutes at times are better than large doses. Larger doses may be repeated every ten to thirty minutes until relief occurs. If no relief develops after two hours or so, the patient may be "epinephrine fast" and necessitate other procedures discussed below. The slow administration of 0.2 to 0.8 cc. of epinephrine solution 1 to 1000 over a period of three to five minutes may be helpful. Rarely, a patient may be allergic to epinephrine and an "Arthus-like" necrosis or ulcer may develop at each site of ingestion. Occasionally, the epinephrine may enter the circulation due to the needle piercing a small arteriole. Then, palpitation, dizziness, severe trembling, and weakness develop, but are rarely if ever serious. If relief occurs from epinephrine, it may be repeated every one to six hours if necessary for weeks, months, or even years without apparent injury. However, such continued symptoms stress the importance of further study of the causative allergies, the gradual control of which will eradicate all or most of the asthmatic symptoms.

Epinephrine in a 1 to 100 or 1 to 50 solution, when vaporized with a proper atomizer and inhaled deep into the bronchial tract, will control most mild recurrent bronchial asthma. The number of deep inhalations of such vapor required to give relief depends on the density of the vapor and the degree of asthma. Such inhalation may be repeated every few minutes, if necessary, until relief occurs. The continuous inhalation of such vapor from an atomizer activated by oxygen or air under pressure until 1 to 2 cc. have been inhaled, has given marked relief in some intractable cases. *Care must be taken not to swallow any drops of this strong epinephrine solution since gastro-intestinal distress and cramping*

8

may result. Therefore, rinsing the mouth after any prolonged or repeated inhalation is recommended.

Epinephrine suspended in oil injected intramuscularly as described by Keeney produces a prolonged epinephrine effect in many cases. Since allergy to peanuts is not uncommon, I have advised that sesame oil be used since allergy to it is extremely rare.

Ephedrine sulphate in ⅜ or ¾ grain capsules, taken by mouth, relieves mild asthmatic symptoms. Since it often produces nervousness and, if repeated often, may produce spasm of the bladder sphincter and urinary retention in men, its use, at times, is contraindicated. When combined with a barbital and in addition with aminophyllin, the nervousness may be eliminated and the action of the ephedrine increased. Recently, enteric coated capsules have been used, so that the action of the ephedrine is delayed three to six hours. These are useful when nocturnal asthma is present. Ephedrine, hypodermically or by inhalation, is not as effective as is epinephrine.

The iodides have long been used for the control of bronchial asthma. Some patients are relieved entirely through such medication, accounting for the relief obtained from many proprietary medicines which usually contain iodides. The saturated solution of potassium or sodium iodide in from 5 to 20 drop doses in water three or four times a day, according to the age of the patient, should be taken until relief occurs. Then, a gradual reduction of dosage is indicated, to be discontinued or resumed according to the symptoms. All patients should be told about idiosyncrasies to iodides. If nasal congestion or a headache develops, or if swelling of the glands under the jaw or a rash or pimples occur, then the iodide should be discontinued. It may be resumed if asthma recurs, in doses which can be tolerated without undue discomfort. The *oral administration of iodides to determine any possible allergy thereto, before they are injected intravenously or instilled* intrabronchially, should be routine.

The inhalation of smoke from the burning powder of stramonium leaves and saltpeter and at times belladonna and lobelia, which are the main ingredients of such proprietary preparations, relieves many patients. However, the same relief is now available from the procedures already outlined, making unnecessary the use of such disagreeable and dirt producing preparations.

Morphine, opiates, and large doses of barbitals should not be used for relief of bronchial asthma. The patient must be alert when asthma is present. Drowsiness or stupor in severe attacks may lead to improper oxygenation of the blood, asphyxia, and at times to death.   This contraindication for morphine is especially justified since the other procedures here described for the relief of symptoms are now available.

Small doses of barbitals may be warranted for sedation only. *Paraldehyde*, moreover, given by rectum, at times, gives very definite relief and is followed by increased mucoid expectoration. The *use of ether in oil, given by rectum*, may be used in selected patients as described in larger textbooks.   The following therapy of severe asthma has displaced the necessity of such ether and oil except in very rare patients.

Patients who continue to have *persistent bronchial asthma* in spite of the above procedures *may be definitely benefited by x-ray therapy* as advised by Maytum.   Such therapy, however, is rarely more than palliative, and the continued study of the causative allergies and therapy directed to their eradication or control are most necessary.

When *severe or intractable bronchial asthma* is present which is associated with great discomfort and possibly cyanosis or evidences of cardiac failure or circulatory collapse, the *patient must be given only foods selected from the elimination diets* as discussed above.   They may have to be in a liquid or soft form.   *Environmental control must be established* as already noted.   The *benefit possible to be obtained from epinephrine, ephedrine, and iodide therapy already recommended must be utilized.*

Patients, however, may fail to obtain relief.   The physician, then, may first try the effect of *aminophyllin $3\frac{1}{2}$ to $7\frac{1}{2}$ grains in solution according to age, given by vein during a two or three minute period*, repeated if necessary one or two times during a twenty-four hour period.   If fluids have not been taken and possible dehydration of the body tissues is present, *glucose solution may be given by vein until adequate fluid can be taken by mouth.*   Such glucose may be in salt solution if the blood chlorides have been depleted and if the oral intake of sodium chloride has been inadequate.   Excessive salt solution, however, may be dangerous.   If the asthmatic symptoms fail to respond, then the *continuous inhalation of 100 per cent oxygen with a Boothby, Lovelace, Bulbulion (B.L.B.) mask*, and if such a mask is not tolerated, oxygen therapy in an oxygen tent would be important.   If relief does not result, then *the inhalation of a mixture of oxygen 20 per cent and helium 80 per cent, preferably with a B.L.B. mask* or in a tent properly constructed for the use of helium gas, would be desirable.   With the continued use of such oxygen therapy, and especially of the helium oxygen inhalation over four to six hours, the severe asthma often ameliorates, mucus begins to be expectorated and the patient responds to epinephrine or aminophyllin therapy.

As relief occurs, the continuance of the elimination diet, environmental control, iodide therapy, and necessary epinephrine therapy are absolutely necessary until symptoms greatly or entirely diminish. Thereafter, the gradual determination of the allergenic foods and the necessity of continued environmental control and hyposensitization therapy, as already discussed in this section, can be made. *Coöperation of the patient over a long period of time,* as emphasized on page 41, is most important whenever bronchial asthma is present.

Bronchoscopy should be done whenever bronchial obstruction from mucus, growths or foreign bodies is suspected. Prickman, recently, has reported benefit from bronchoscopy in bronchial constriction due to chronic or intermittent localized inflammations. *Non-specific therapy* with intravenous typhoid vaccine and *neoarsphenamine* in some cases of chronic asthma, especially if spirochetes are in the sputum, is discussed in the larger text of the writer. Finally, the use *psychotherapy* is most necessary in certain patients especially when psychogenic asthma is suspected.

SEASONAL AND PERENNIAL NASAL ALLERGY
(HAY FEVER)

When the allergy affects the mucosa of the nasal passages and, at times, of the sinuses, so-called hay fever results. *Pollen allergy* produces seasonal symptoms in the spring, summer, or fall months according to the pollens which cause sensitization. Here, in California, where pollen continues in the air throughout the year, perennial nasal allergy from pollen may occur. Some patients are sensitive to practically all pollens so that symptoms begin with the first grass and tree pollination, and extend into the late fall when the frosts begin. Others only have symptoms when one type of pollen is in the air, notably ragweed pollen. Frequently the ocular tissues are affected, and bronchial asthma or bronchitis may also occur. Some patients, moreover, have allergic dermatitis and, rarely, gastro-intestinal symptoms from such pollen allergy.

Nasal allergy, moreover, may arise from all the *various animal emanation and dust allergens, and from miscellaneous allergens,* including orris root, karaya gum, pyrethrum, kapok, cottonseed, and spores of fungi already described in the section on bronchial asthma, and especially in Chapter III. Such inhalants are prone to cause perennial nasal allergy or symptoms in certain environments when specific allergens are inhaled.

Food allergy is a common cause of nasal allergy. Usually, the symptoms are perennial unless some seasonal food is responsible. Moreover, the *symptoms from common foods are usually worse in the winter months and better in the summer period and away from the ocean, as is true of bronchial asthma due to foods.*

Bacterial allergy is a very rare cause of nasal allergy. Vaccine therapy is rarely beneficial. Gradually, surgical therapy on the nose, both for nasal allergy and bronchial asthma, is becoming less frequent. Its indications are discussed below.

Nasal allergy, due to inhalants and especially to pollens, is characterized by sneezing, watery or mucoid discharge from the nose, watering, burning, and redness of the eyes, varying degrees of nasal congestion and blocking which may be especially bad at night, and itching of the nose, eyes, and, at times, of the throat, nasopharynx, palate, Eustachian tubes, and sometimes of the skin of the face and neck. *Nasal allergy, due to food, is more often associated with marked congestion, blocking and loss of smell.* Sneezing may be severe and paroxysmal. *Itching* which is so frequent in inhalant allergy, *may be nearly or completely absent.*

Chronic nasal allergy especially when it also involves the eustachian tubes and middle ear may impair hearing and predispose to tinnitus. Tendency to recurrent otitis media in childhood moreover may be increased by uncontrolled nasal or aural allergy.

X-ray studies of the sinuses and, especially, of the maxillary sinuses, may show opacities, either due to thickened mucosa and accumulated mucus in such sinuses purely due to localized mucous membrane allergy therein, or due to absence of aëration because of the closure of the ostia, due again to allergic edema in the mucosa. *Formerly, the serious mistake was made of assuming infection in such antra and sinuses merely because opacities were demonstrated by x-ray or transillumination.*

At present, the *microscopic examination of the nasal mucus* and that obtained from sinuses suspected of infection or allergy is an important diagnostic test, as proposed especially by Hansel. The secretions are smeared on a glass slide, stained with Wright's or Giemsa's solution and searched for eosinophiles and for pus cells. Clumps of eosinophiles indicate allergy; pus cells favor infection. Both types suggest allergy and infection. Absent eosinophiles even on several occasions do not rule out allergy.

If allergy is suspected the *patient must be examined and skin tested as recommended in bronchial asthma. Food* and *inhalant* allergy must be studied and treated as described. Proper use of elimination *diets* when food allergy is at all possible is most important. *Environmental control*, the use of antigens containing various inhalants indicated by history and skin testing and the use of properly prepared *house dust and other types of dust antigens*, as discussed in the section on Bronchial Asthma, are most necessary when such inhalant allergy is possible. *Orris root* as a cause of nasal allergy must be remembered and allergen-free cosmetics and orris root hyposensitization must be used. *Feather, pyrethrum, kapok, and cottonseed allergies* are common causes. For a more complete consideration of the details of diagnosis and treatment, the reader should consult the larger texts, such as that of the writer and others listed on page 257.

Surgery on the nose and sinuses for the relief of nasal allergy should only be done after an adequate allergic study has been made and proper anti-allergic treatment carried out for several weeks or even months. Polyps in the nose itself which obstruct breathing may need early removal. When marked deviation of the septum is present, and after allergy has been brought under control, the correction of such deviation may be advisable. As noted above, antra and sinuses should never be operated upon merely because an opacity is demonstrated. If actual pus is shown by microscopic examination, and evidences of acute inflammation of the antra or other sinuses are present, then proper washing or surgery would be in order. *Too often in the past, operations done on allergic antra or sinuses have led to secondary infections which have, in turn, necessitated further surgery.* Such superimposed infections in sinuses still affected with unrecognized and uncontrolled allergy have led to so-called chronic sinusitis, further surgery, varying degrees of invalidism, and often to other clinical complications.

Temporary relief from symptoms of nasal allergy can be obtained at times from the instillation or the spraying into the nose of 1 per cent ephedrine in salt solution, or of 0.25 per cent neosynephrine. The ingestion of ephedrine $\frac{3}{8}$ or $\frac{3}{4}$ grain or the use of ephedrine combined with a barbital may give relief. At times, the use of potassium iodide, as advised in bronchial asthma, may be helpful. The use of epinephrine 1 to 1000 hypodermically may also be indicated. All of these, however, give very temporary help, and the patient's discomfort is not satisfactorily relieved until the allergenic causes are discovered and gradually controlled.

Atopic Dermatitis (Eczema) and Contact Dermatitis (Eczema).—*Atopic dermatitis or eczema is due to blood borne allergens absorbed from ingested foods or drugs, inhalants of all types entering the nasal or bronchial tracts, or from bacterial, fungoid, or parasitical* *infections in various parts of the body.* Positive urticarial or hive-like skin reactions, a positive family history of allergy and the so-called Prausnitz-Küstner reacting bodies in the blood are usually present in such atopic patients. *Thus, most infantile eczema, eczema in young children and many adults are of this type arising from blood-borne allergens. The dermatitis results from allergic reactions in the sensitized tissues of the capillaries in the lower layers of the true skin.* Because of increased vascular permeability, fluid exudes, forming areas of edema with resultant minute papules or vesicles. These gradually increase in size and become palpable through the epidermis. Itching usually is intense and scratching and rubbing of the skin may break open the multitudinous vesicles with resultant oozing of serous fluid. Later, crusting, thickening, and lichenification of the skin occur. Oozing may gradually cease but scaling, thickening and itching of the skin continues. At times, minute and diffuse papules instead of vesicles form, and scaling, thickening, and itching occur without associated oozing and crusting. Because of the scratching and rubbing of the skin, excoriations practically always are present in varying degrees.

Infantile eczema is usually atopic in type, being due to blood-borne allergens, especially from ingested foods. Nursing infants may be allergic to food allergens in the mother's milk. When foods allergenic to the baby are eliminated from the mother's diet, the nursing infant's eczema may improve and disappear. Milk and eggs in particular and cereal grains, fish, and certain fruits are common causes.

As age increases, blood-borne allergens from various inhalants, such as feathers, wool, kapok, cottonseed, silk, animal emanations, other miscellaneous inhalants including house and environmental dusts, and pollens, may cause such eczema though *food allergy still remains the major cause through infancy.*

Atopic dermatitis in children after the first year and especially in older children and young adults *arises more frequently from inhalant allergy.* When the dermatitis occurs in the spring, summer, or fall months, pollen allergy even when skin reactions are negative, must be suspected. When the lesions decrease in the summer and are worse in the fall, winter, and spring, environmental allergens and food allergy, as noted on page 58, must be studied.

Skin testing in infants should only be done by the scratch test with ingested foods and with encountered inhalant allergens. *Older children may be tested* with a larger number of food, inhalant, dust, and especially pollen allergens by the scratch test. Those inhalant allergens under suspicion which have failed to react by the scratch test (see page 24) may be tested intradermally. *Adults should be thoroughly tested* as has been suggested for the asthmatic patient. The fallibility of the skin test, as discussed in Chapter I, must always be in mind.

For the diagnosis of food allergy, the use of elimination diets is necessary in practically every case. At present, many poor results in atopic dermatitis or eczema, especially in infants, but also throughout life, in the writer's opinion, are due to the dependence on test negative diets and the failure to use adequate diet trial with elimination diets. For infants, a special elimination diet is detailed on page 183. For children over one year of age, another diet is available on page 184. For older children and adults, the various elimination diets in amounts according to age and caloric requirements are detailed in Chapter V. The time necessary for such diet trial, the necessity of absolute strictness and coöperation, and the other precautions stressed throughout this book must be remembered at all times if food allergy is to receive proper consideration. In infancy, especially, it is necessary that adequate protein intake is assured and that anemia and hypoproteinemia do not occur. Edema from such nutritional damage has been observed.

For the study of inhalant allergy, environmental control, as discussed in the section on Bronchial Asthma, *in addition to the adequate history and indicated skin testing, may be necessary.*

When food allergy is present, the foods may have to be excluded for several months or even years before tolerance is established. *When inhalant allergy is active,* environmental control may suffice or hyposensitization, as discussed in the section on Asthma, may be required. *When pollen allergy is present,* treatment often must be given with very dilute antigens, since such therapy should never increase or exaggerate the dermatitis. *Co-seasonal daily therapy* may be necessary for several weeks until definite improvement occurs. (See page 41.)

Seborrhea, pyogenic and at times fungus infections of the skin may complicate atopic dermatitis and may be mistaken for the latter. Moreover, *the naturally dry, ichthyotic skin which scales and itches* must always be recognized and such patients should not be treated for assumed allergy. In infancy, especially, *seborrhea of the skin, particularly when the scalp is involved, must be properly treated.* Scratching must be prevented as much as possible and indicated dermatological therapy at all times must be used.

Contact dermatitis or eczema *is due to a sensitization of the superficial epidermal cells to various contactant substances.* In contrast, atopic dermatitis, as stated above, arises from localized allergic reactivity in the vascular bed in the deeper layers of the skin from blood-borne allergens. The mechanism of contact dermatitis with the many possible causes and its diagnosis have been discussed already on page 99.

When *such contact dermatitis* is severe as occurs from poison ivy or poison oak and from many other vegetations and contact substances, *it is often called dermatitis venenata. Temporary relief,* especially when oozing is present, is best obtained with moist compresses of boric acid solution, dilute Burow's solution, or with hot or cold salt solution or water. A 2 or 3 per cent tannic acid solution may relieve itching and prevent spreading. As the dermatitis becomes drier, calamine lotion with 0.5 per cent phenol or with liquor carbonis detergens, and later various ointments, as recommended by dermatologists, may be helpful. When the dermatitis is due to an oil or resin from some prevalent plant or weed such as ragweed, cocklebur, helenium, or mugwort, it is often necessary for the patient to leave the area where such vegetation is, until the dermatitis improves, and until the oil leaves the air. Contact allergy from various substances encountered in the home, working or recreational environments, especially in the industries, necessitates the prevention of all possibilities of contact with the allergenic substance. At times, it means a change of occupation.

Hyposensitization to the oils and resins of various vegetations which cause contact dermatitis has been reported by various procedures. In poison ivy and oak, dilutions of the oil and resin have been given intramuscularly and by mouth with varying success. It would seem unwise to administer it during the actual attack, but only for prevention. Dilutions of oils of the leaves of various vegetations which produce contact dermatitis, especially of ragweed, cocklebur, helenium and the sages have been used. Results from intramuscular therapy have not been encouraging. Shelmire, however, observed some protection, varying according to the patient, when the diluted plant oil was given orally before the seasonal dermatitis began, first with increasing doses of a 1 to 100 dilution, then with similar doses of a 1 to 50 and later a 1 to 25 dilution. The dose must vary according to the patient's tolerance. The oil is given in a gelatin capsule to prevent dermatitis of the lips and soreness of the mouth and throat. *Further experience with such plant oils will gradually determine their therapeutic value.*

Much evidence points to the benefit of hyposensitization with the specific pollens of the weed, plant, or tree rather than with the leaf, or pollen oil of which the patient gives a contact reaction. Several patients with contact reactions to sagebrush, mugwort, and cocklebur have been entirely or nearly completely relieved with prolonged pre-seasonal pollen therapy and a few have been helped by co-seasonal therapy with such pollen antigens as described on page 40.   Such relief may be due to small amounts of the specific oil in the pollen, though most pollens are cleaned with ether. Favorable results have also been reported with hyposensitization with ragweed pollen antigens in patients with contact reactions to the ragweed oil.

Hyposensitization with various dyes, chemicals of all types, lacquers, and the many other substances discussed on page 53 has not been accomplished.   At present, the removal of the patient from all possibilities of contact with such causative allergenic substances must be depended upon for relief.

Urticaria and Angioneurotic Edema.— *Urticaria or hives are due to localized allergy in the capillaries and small arterioles in the skin, and angioneurotic edema or acute circumscribed edema arises from such allergy in the larger blood-vessels of the skin and subcutaneous tissues.*   The lymphatics may also be affected.   Increased permeability of these vascular tissues allows exudation of fluid and consequent edema, the resultant hives or swellings depending on the degree and extent of the allergic reaction.   The evanescent and wandering nature of the affections is due to increased allergy in certain vascular areas with consequent desensitization or refractoriness resulting in inability of those particular areas to react for varying periods of time.

It is important to remember that *urticaria has been observed in the mucous membranes of the mouth, pharynx, esophagus, and bronchial tract and that it probably also occurs in the mucosa of the gastro-intestinal tract.*

Angioneurotic edema usually involves the skin and subcutaneous tissues of the face, lips, neck, hands, and feet, and less frequently any other area.   It often affects the *tongue and throat.*   When *laryngeal edema* occurs, suffocation and even death may result. Such swellings may occur in the *gastro-intestinal tract* or other abdominal organs, producing pain, acute digestive symptoms, occasionally causing temporary intestinal obstruction, so-called phantom tumors, and swellings with cramping and varying distress in localized areas of the colon, sigmoid, or rectum.   Angioneurotic edema may also occur *in the brain or spinal cord* and their membranes, causing symptoms of brain or cord tumors, in the *urogenital tract* or in the *lungs*, producing evidences of a transient pneumonia. When such swelling occurs *in the joint tissues, so-called intermittent hydrarthrosis may occur.* The skin and subcutaneous tissues, however, are the areas of predilection.

These allergic manifestations most frequently arise from food allergy. Fruits and fish are common causes of urticaria and less frequently of angioneurotic edema. Those foods excluded from the elimination diets also must always be suspected and the realization that any food or condiment, including those in the elimination diets, may cause these allergic manifestations, must be remembered. *Drugs of many types must always be considered.*

Bacterial allergy from foci of infection, especially in the teeth and gums, tonsils, prostate, and anal fistulæ, and less commonly in the sinuses, gall-bladder, appendix, and even from the bacterial flora in the membranes of the nasopharyngeal or bronchial tissues and in the gastro-intestinal tract and diverticulæ, requires adequate study. *Other infectant allergy from epidermophytosis or other fungus infections or monilia,* especially in the colon, or from *animal parasites* in the gastro-intestinal tract or other body tissues, must be in mind. Urticaria may also arise from one or more *bites of mosquitoes, mites, bees, yellow jackets, wasps, and bedbugs.* The fact that *flea bites* produce an eruption simulating urticaria and that generalized urticaria from one or two flea bites may occur, is necessary to remember. *Inhalant allergy,* especially from pollens, but also from dusts, animal emanations, spores of fungi, and other miscellaneous inhalants discussed in Chapter III causes urticaria in occasional patients. *Physical allergy,* especially to cold and heat, must be remembered as primary or secondary causes in few sufferers. *Neuroses* are thought by some students to be responsible for these and other manifestations of allergy, as noted on page 108. It is my opinion that nervousness rarely is primarily the cause, but that it may activate underlying allergies as do physical stimuli.

Dermographia.—Dermographia is characterized by easy welting of the skin when pressure, stroking or striking the skin occurs. It seems that a rapid release of histamine-like substances may be responsible. The writer thinks, however, that most of these patients have a long-standing underlying or potential allergy and that its gradual and proper control will reduce and, at times, eradicate the dermographia. This is discussed at this point since it is often confused with true urticaria.

The determination of the allergenic causes as usual requires a carefully recorded history, as suggested on page 19, from which the probable type of allergy can often be surmised. Positive skin reactions to foods productive of *urticaria and angioneurotic edema* are especially difficult to obtain by the scratch test except for those large reactions which occur when foods produce marked symptoms soon after the ingestion of the food. In such cases, the patient usually is aware of his specific allergies and the positive skin reaction is superfluous. Remembering that the negative skin reaction does not rule out food allergy, and that positive reactions, especially by the intradermal test, are often indicative of no clinical allergy, it is, nevertheless, advisable to test the patient by the scratch method as recommended on page 23 with all important ingestant allergens. Tests with all important inhalants, including a few pollens, with subsequent intradermal testing with important inhalants which have failed to react by the scratch method, are also advisable in most patients with these manifestations, especially if inhalant allergy is suggested by the history. The choice of such inhalant allergens, the technic and interpretation of the test are discussed in Chapter II.

As in most patients suspected of food allergy, because of the fallibility of the skin tests, trial diet with elimination diets is advisable.   Usually fruit should be excluded from the initial elimination diet in these cases because of the frequency of fruit allergy as a cause of these manifestations. Menus for such fruit-free elimination diets are detailed on pages 171 to 175. Allergy to fruits, either one or two, or, often seemingly to all fruits may exist. Sensitization to allergens in uncooked vegetables may also occur and additional allergy to tomato may exist. After relief has occurred, the gradual addition, first of cooked or canned fruits in the routine elimination diets may be tried. As in all food sensitive patients, *the manifestations may continue to recur decreasingly for days or even weeks, even when the causative allergens have been entirely eliminated.* This is probably due, as stated on page 141, to the persistence of the food allergens in the body tissues, especially in those of the shock organs, for varying periods of time. At times, such allergy to fruits may continue for weeks, months, and in a few patients, for years. With their exclusion, additional vitamin C from 25 to 100 mg. by mouth should be given. As discussed on page 171, if allergy to cevitamic acid (vitamin C) also exists, then those vegetables which contain most of this vitamin as discussed on page 203 should be stressed in the diet. After tolerance for fruits is determined, other foods in the elimination diets and all additional foods can gradually be added as advised on page 145.

When bacterial allergy is present, complete eradication of the foci of infection is imperative. In some cases, these bacterial allergens also persist in the body tissues for weeks or months, accounting for continued or recurrent symptoms. Proper vaccine therapy, discussed on page 103, may be necessary. Allergy from the decay in several teeth apparently caused urticaria in one patient. The eradication of infectants of other types described above is necessary for relief. Hyposensitization, *when allergy to fungus allergens exists,* may be necessary. *Relief from hypersensitivity to various insect bites,* including those of fleas, is possible with specific allergenic treatment as formerly noted on page 104.

When inhalant sensitizations are possible causes, as evidenced by history or skin reactions, hyposensitization with properly prepared antigens, as discussed in Chapter III, becomes necessary. The final diagnosis of such inhalant allergy as a cause may depend on the results of such hyposensitization.

Other less common causes of these manifestations need the special attention advised in larger texts and in the literature of allergy.

Until the allergenic causes of urticaria and angioneurotic edema are determined and eliminated or controlled with proper therapy, *the relief of the pruritus and a reduction of the swellings often are urgent.* This is especially true if the swellings are in the larynx threatening respiration, in the tongue and throat preventing adequate nourishment, or in the gastro-intestinal tract causing severe pain, vomiting or other symptoms. Epinephrine 1 to 1000 from 0.2 to 0.8 cc. doses hypodermically according to age and repeated every ten to sixty minutes for several days as necessary for relief is of most benefit. The inhalation of 1 to 100 epinephrine as described on page 113 fails to relieve hives or cutaneous allergic swellings. The oral or intravenous administration of calcium is of no value and peptone therapy along with urotherapy advised a few years ago is useless. Autohemotherapy, likewise, has failed in practically all cases. Recently, the oral administration of histaminase, a ferment which breaks down histamine, has been advised. Relief which occurs in a few cases is not permanent until the allergenic causes are found. Alexander and others recently have advised histamine by vein and subcutaneously in chronic allergy especially in urticaria. Its success in a few cases warrants its continued trial. The hypodermic administration of histaminase has been advised. Recently, Arthus-like necroses have been reported from such injections and its value is still to be demonstrated.

The itching and burning of urticaria are alleviated at times by *local therapy.* Bathing in warm water to which a cup of soda and of cornstarch are added with subsequent patting of the skin with a towel until fairly dry may be repeated several times a day. Cold or iced compresses at times are helpful. Various lotions containing small amounts of phenol, menthol, calamine or other antipruritic agents, as recommended by textbooks on dermatology, especially in Sulzberger's recent book, may be used.

The *urticaria of serum sickness* requires therapy as outlined above. Reports indicate that histaminase is especially helpful. Its oral administration for a week or ten days after serum therapy might be advisable to prevent possible serum sickness. The precautions advisable in the administration of serum, especially to allergic patients, are discussed on page 226.

Generalized edema or extensive edema of large parts of the body may arise from allergy and may last for a day or so or persist with variations for long periods of time. When such edema occurs, an increase of from 5 to 15 pounds in weight may result in a few days. Such edema may continue until the causative allergens cease operating or may disappear when the allergic reactivity is exhausted and refractoriness to the causative allergens arise. Then, in varying periods, as the allergy in the tissues mounts, a recurrence of the edema results. Such generalized edema is often associated with drowsiness, mental confusion, and fatigue due in part to cerebral edema. Headache and a low grade fever may also occur.

Food allergy and occasional bacterial allergy are the most frequent causes. Inhalant allergy should also be in mind, though the writer has never seen it operative in such generalized edema.

The diagnosis and treatment of this syndrome are similar to that already discussed for urticaria.

Acne.—The beneficial results from elimination diets in acne vulgaris obtained by the writer since 1931 were discussed in his textbook in 1937. White in 1934 and Cormia in 1940 reported similar benefit with elimination diets. Such results naturally have suggested food allergy as a possible cause. This etiology is also indicated by the rapid increase of acne after the addition of specific foods, especially of milk, egg and chocolate. Allergic etiology, moreover, is suggested by acne due to iodides in susceptible patients and by seasonal acne from pollen.

For years, it has been known that "rich foods" increase acne. Recently good results in acne similar to those from elimination diets have been reported by Sutton with low-fat diets. Milk, butter, chocolate, bacon, fats of meats, oils and shortenings are excluded. He attributes acne to pustular epidermal lipoidosis due to improper metabolism of lipoids and recommends thyroid extract when hypothyroidism exists, to increase lipoid utilization. In about 10 per cent of his patients with acne, he also uses a low-carotene diet when rosy yellow or xanthoma-like lesions occur.

Whether food allergy or impaired lipoid metabolism explains the good results obtained with the elimination diets and the fat-poor diet is impossible to decide at present. Gradually the rôle of both of these possible causes will be determined. For the present we continue to use the elimination diet, preferably the cereal-free type. Fats are reduced to a minimum providing adequate calories in the other foods will insure a satisfactory weight. The possible production of acne by iodized salt is still considered and the ability to tolerate it as suggested by Sutton when thyroid is given is being studied. When reduced resistance to skin organisms is shown by definite pustules, autogenous vaccines are used. Dermatological therapy including x-ray treatment is reserved for the minority of patients who do not respond satisfactorily or rapidly enough to the diet manipulation.

Miscellaneous Manifestations.—The probability that *lupus erythematosus may be due to allergy* to various ingestant, inhalant or bacterial allergens, including occasionally tuberculin allergy, has been stated by various students. A thorough study of a group of these patients needs to be done to obtain more evidence of the possible rôle of allergy in this disease.

As stated on page 138, *erythema nodosum* is probably due to vascular allergy and the other *so-called erythemas* are practically all due to an allergic state. The fact that the *eruptions of the contagious diseases* are the result of specific allergy to the infectants concerned must be here recalled.

GASTRO–INTESTINAL ALLERGY

Allergy may cause reactions in the mouth, throat, esophagus, stomach, intestines, rectum, and anus, according to which areas are especially sensitized. Other manifestations of allergy as described in this chapter may also occur in the same patient.

Oral and Pharyngeal Allergy.—*Physicians and especially dentists must recognize the allergic lesions on the lips, in the mouth and throat.* Cheilitis, characterized by erythema, edema, vesiculation, oozing, and crusting of the lips, may arise from contact allergy to ingredients in mouth washes, toothpastes, dental floss, cigarettes, foods, contacted metallic or lacquered articles, or medicines. Dyes in lipstick, especially tetrabromfluorescin, and azo dyes, often cause cheilitis.   Perfume, polishes for nails, the essential oils or hexylresorcinol in toothpastes may be responsible.   Patch tests with suspected substances as described on page 99 may indicate the specific cause.   *Perleche,* characterized by thickening, desquamation, maceration, or fissuring of the corners of the mouth, may be due to food and at times, to contact allergy.   Riboflavin deficiency may also cause these lip lesions.   *Hives or angioneurotic edema,* due to food and less often to drug or bacterial allergy, may affect the lips.   *Recurrent cold sores* may be due to food or drug allergy.   As noted on page 51, allergy is responsible for *swelling from insect bites.*

Inflammation of the oral mucosa (*stomatitis*), of the gums (*gingivitis*) or of the tongue (*glossitis*), may arise from food or drug allergy as from infection or irritations from carious teeth or poorly fitting caps or dentures.   Drug allergy may produce various types of oral lesions.   The acetanalide, antipyrin and the barbital and halogen drugs must be remembered.   Phenolphthalein, particularly, may produce blebs, vesicles, erosions in the oral mucosa, burning and tingling of the tongue.   *Pricking or burning of the tongue or a metallic taste may be due to allergy.*   Swellings of the tongue, gums, oral mucosa, or pharynx may arise from food allergy.   The *"geographic tongue"* may be due to allergy, especially to food.

The burning, tingling, and congestive lesions which arise from the *galvanic reaction between gold, nickel and amalgam in dentures and fillings* must be recalled in our discussion of oral allergy.

Aphthæ or canker sores are usually due to food and less often to drug, denture, or bacterial allergies.   When secondarily infected, serious inflammations may arise.   The frequency of food allergy, especially to fruits in the etiology of canker sores, requires the use of trial elimination diets in the study of such cases as described in this book.   Other types of allergy noted above must receive attention.

Vulcanite and other synthetic dentures may produce allergic stomatitis or gingivitis with redness, vesiculation, blebs, excoriations, cracking, and oozing.   Allergy to a single dye, to mercury, rubber, or other mineral substances may occur.   Patch tests with all ingredients may show the specific cause.   Allergy to hecolite with positive patch tests on the skin is not uncommon.

Agranulocytosis, producing ulcerative, necrotic stomatitis, leucopenia, and an absence of the granular cells in the blood, is probably due to allergy in the blood forming cells of the bone-marrow. Amidopyrine, especially, and also arsphenamine, gold salts, cincophen, dinitrophenol and sulphanilamide have been responsible.

Oral, as well as cutaneous, lesions to anesthetics, such as novocaine, procaine, butyn, and apothesine in patient, dentist, and assistant, must be remembered. Other drugs, antiseptics, and mouth washes used in dental work must be suspected.

Orthodontia often becomes necessary in children because of nasal allergy to foods or inhalants which cause blocking of the nose, a high palate, a narrow and protruding upper dental arch.

A *coated tongue and halitosis* may be due to food allergy, causing localized allergy in the stomach or intestines with resultant mild or marked reversed peristalsis. *Postnasal mucus, causing throat clearing and hacking of mucus,* may also cause coated tongue and is often due to food or inhalant allergies. *Localized allergy in the pharynx* may produce recurrent irritation, congestion, or soreness, often mistaken for actual infection.

In *the esophagus,* allergy may produce swellings or spasms. It may cause some cases of globus hystericus. Spasm of the lower end of the esophagus (cardiospasm) may arise from allergy impairing proper entrance of food or fluid into the stomach.

Gastric Allergy.—Gastric allergy, associated with mucous membrane congestion or inflammation or smooth muscle spasm, may give rise to burning or pyrosis, cramping, belching, regurgitation, distention, and nausea in varying degrees and combinations. When pyloric spasm or impaired peristalsis occurs, vomiting may arise. The *possibility that peptic ulcer may arise as canker-like lesions from allergy* is suggested by the clinical experiences of allergists.

Intestinal Allergy.—Allergy in various parts of the *small intestine* may result in similar symptoms associated with localized cramping or pain in other parts of the abdomen and diarrhea. *Colonic allergy* may produce localized pain or soreness in the cecum, ascending transverse or descending colon, in the sigmoid or rectum. *Diarrhea* or *constipation* may occur. *Mucous colitis* is often due to allergy, having been described in the past as "asthma of the bowel." Long-standing constipation, the *so-called irritable bowel, distended colon or a sensation of incomplete bowel evacuation* and so-called tenesmus may be due to allergy and be relieved by the elimination of allergenic foods, rarely of drugs, and occasionally by hyposensitization therapy with inhalants, especially with pollens.

Ulcerative colitis, the etiology of which has long been uncertain, may be primarily due to allergy. Mackie particularly, in 1939, concluded that food allergy was important in 65 per cent of his series of 67 cases. In this group, it appears that the possibilities of trial diet with various elimination diets were not entirely exhausted.

9

The etiological rôle of food allergy in this disease has also been emphasized in several cases studied by the writer in the last four years. It is possible that the colon may be the site of localized allergy to food or possibly other types of allergy, including bacterial allergy, and that *allergic inflammation with canker-like lesions* of varying degree may be the initial manifestations. Later, secondary infection with resultant cellulitis, formation of scar tissue and extension of ulcerations may lead to the advanced lesions. Thus, these patients should be studied with diet trial while other possible causes are being considered. The use of adequate vitamins, the administration of liver extract parenterally, attention to anemia and necessary surgery in advanced cases, as stressed recently by Cave, are most important. For diet trial, the fruit-free elimination diets, prepared in a liquid or puréed form, as noted on page 171, should first be prescribed in most cases of this disease. More restricted supplemental diets described on page 181 may be advisable.

As stated on page 122, localized edema in various parts of the intestine may cause *severe abdominal pain and even signs of intestinal obstruction*, leading to unnecessary surgery. So-called *"cecal and appendiceal allergy"* has also been responsible for many appendicial operations. However, when surgery is definitely indicated, it should never be postponed. *Allergy and infection may coexist in the same patient.*

Localized allergy undoubtedly affects the liver in varying degrees and areas. The decreased hepatic function and flow of bile arising from such possible allergy are difficult to measure. Allergic congestion and spasm in the gall-bladder and biliary tract may give rise to symptoms of biliary colic or gall-bladder disease, making allergy one of the necessary diagnostic considerations in upper abdominal symptomatology. Such allergy may also affect the pancreas, but this is difficult to determine.

In infancy, much *colic* is due to food allergy often to milk and less frequently to eggs, wheat, and fruits and other foods. *Bleeding from the bowel or melena,* due to increased permeability in the capillaries of the bowel mucosa, may arise from food allergy. Food allergy has also been responsible for *pylorospasm* in certain infants as reported in the literature. *Other gastro-intestinal symptoms described above* may also occur in infants and young children. *Recurrent or cyclic vomiting, especially, is frequently due to food allergy.* It is often associated with headache and is a forerunner of sick headaches or migraine in later life.

Finally, *spasm in the anal muscles and especially pruritus or itching around the anus may be due to allergy.* Such pruritus ani necessitates a thorough study of possible food allergy and a consideration of allergy to bacteria and to fungi, particularly to monilia in the intestinal tract.

The study of the patient for possible allergy requires the same carefully recorded history, the limited information from skin testing, and especially the use of diet trial with various elimination diets as already outlined in the previous sections of this chapter. In gastro-intestinal allergy, sensitization to several or even all fruits as in urticaria is not infrequent. This may require the initial use of a fruit-free elimination diet (see page 171) or the use of such a diet after the routine elimination diets with or without cereals have been used for an adequate period. Supplemental diets as described on page 181 may be necessary in patients suspected of food allergy who do not respond to the routine elimination diets. Drug allergies, the occasional bacterial and pollen allergies as causes of gastro-intestinal symptoms must be kept in mind.

For the temporary relief of acute symptoms, while the possible causes are being determined, the use of epinephrine as discussed under bronchial asthma may be helpful. The use of a puréed, liquid or soft diet containing the foods in the selected elimination diet may be necessary, especially if diarrhea, mucous colitis or an irritable bowel is present, as discussed on page 152. The use of histaminase, calcium, and other non-specific therapy has been of no value in this type of allergy.

All patients suspected of allergy, and especially those with gastro-intestinal symptoms, must have *careful physical, laboratory, and x-ray studies.* Actual pathology must not be overlooked. *Absent hydrochloric acid in the stomach or parasites in the bowel* must be recognized since symptoms suggesting possible allergy may arise therefrom. Careful study of possible *vitamin deficiencies from inadequate diets* for months or years is imperative. It is most important to recognize the *nervous indigestion so well emphasized by Alvarez* which occurs in the introspective, neurotic, unstable person who even may be suffering from a mild or actual psychosis. The presence of *hypothyroidism* or *hypogonadism in women and men* must be discovered and treated with proper hormonal therapy. These are a few of the diseased states, more fully discussed in the writer's larger text and in others by various allergists and internists which must be considered in the differential diagnosis of a patient suffering with possible gastro-intestinal allergy.

ALLERGIC MIGRAINE, SICK HEADACHES AND RECURRENT VOMITING

Vaughan, Balyeat, the writer, and other allergists have stressed the allergic etiology of many cases of migraine and sick headache for the last fifteen years. *That allergy also causes much cyclic vomiting with or without headache* in childhood is noted on page 139. The elimination of allergenic foods gives good or excellent relief in approximately 60 to 70 per cent of all such patients and it is probable with perfect coöperation of the patient and the thorough use of elimination diets, as described in this volume, a larger number of patients would be relieved.*

As in all symptoms which at times are due to allergy, *it is most important to recognize all other pathology in these patients*, utilizing proper histories, physical examinations, and laboratory studies. The ocular and nasal headaches, those arising from disturbances in the digestive and biliary functions and from chronic diseases other than allergy must be kept in mind. In such differential diagnosis, however, allergy needs constant consideration.

It is impossible to be certain whether *the allergic reaction produces edema and congestion of the meninges, or whether arterial spasm with possible increased vascular permeability and edema of adjacent cerebral tissue is responsible.* The allergy is certainly localized in varying areas of the brain or the meninges in different patients, accounting for the occurrence of ocular symptoms, of disturbances in hearing or smell, or of paresthesias and pareses, according to the localization of the reaction in the brain. The *cyclic recurrence* of the symptoms is characteristic of allergy, especially to foods as noted on page 56. Many of these patients have *reflex gastro-intestinal symptoms*. Nausea, vomiting and other abdominal symptoms may be due to concomitant allergy in the gastro-intestinal tract.

Whereas food allergy is the most common cause of allergic migraine and headache, *inhalant allergy of different types occasionally is responsible.* Therefore, the history must be taken as outlined on page 56 with all types of allergy in mind. Skin testing with food allergens by the scratch method may be routine, though little helpful information can be expected in the majority of cases. Scratch and intradermal testing with important inhalants should be done whenever any indication of possible inhalant allergy exists. The proper evaluation of the negative and positive skin tests as discussed on page 13 must be remembered.

* Allergic menstrual headaches are discussed on page 108.

For the study of possible food allergy, elimination diets, as described in Chapter V, *should be properly used for adequate periods. Nutrition, as stressed in this volume, must be protected.* The time necessary for such diet trial and for an eventual building of tolerance to allergenic foods is discussed on page 141. When inhalant allergy is probable, the diagnostic and therapeutic recommendations outlined in the section on Bronchial Asthma must be followed.

While the various causes of migraine and recurrent sick-headaches are being studied and diet trial is progressing, the *attacks themselves usually can be relieved with ergotamine tartrate*, 0.25 to 0.5 mg. given hypodermically and repeated if necessary in two or three hours. The resultant discomfort may contraindicate its use. The prolonged use of ergotamine tartrate may produce gangrene of the extremities, especially in patients with vascular disease. *Its use, moreover, seems to postpone the attack, and a more frequent use of the drug often becomes necessary. Habit formation is apparent in some patients.* The oral administration of from 1 to 3 mg. before an attack may be helpful. Epinephrine, 1 to 1000, in doses of 8 to 15 minims, given hypodermically, slowly over a period of three to five minutes, may give relief.

Alvarez especially has advised against overwork, excitement and worry in these patients. *Psychotherapy* may be advisable. Alvarez has also used the *inhalation of* 100 *per cent oxygen* by the B.L.B. mask with benefit to migraine. The relief afforded by *acetyl salicylic acid, antipyrin, or phenacetin* should be obtained. *Codein* in from ½ to 1 grain doses alone or with the above drugs is helpful at times. *Barbitals, bromides*, and *chloral hydrate for sedation* may be advisable. Some of these patients are benefited by saline cathartics or by bile salts with or without phenolphthalein or by colonic flushings or enemas. Such relief occurs at times in those who later are found affected with food allergy. Bacterial allergy from colonic organisms might also be suggested by such relief from enemas. *The writer would again stress the frequency of food allergy in migraine and recurrent sick headaches.*

ALLERGIC TOXEMIA

Food allergy and, less often, pollen allergy, may produce drowsiness, stupor, inability to concentrate, fatigue, and exhaustion, probably due to a cerebral edema. It is often present in patients with allergic migraine and sick headaches and usually occurs when a generalized edema with sudden increases in weight are present, as discussed on page 126. A *low grade fever*, at times recurring on and off for months or years, may be due to uncontrolled chronic allergy.

Other manifestations of allergy may be present. Nasal congestion, watery discharge, and sneezing may arise due to the same allergic reaction in the nasal and sinusal tissues which is causing the nearby cerebral edema. Generalized aching in muscles and joints and chilling of the body, especially when the allergic reaction becomes intensified, may be present, probably due to a generalized allergic tissue reactivity in addition to that in the brain.

When food allergy is suspected, a study similar to that suggested in the discussion of allergic migraine is necessary. Pollen toxemia, usually associated with hay fever, asthma, or allergic dermatitis, must be treated as described under Bronchial Asthma.

A complete physical and laboratory examination must recognize all other possible causes of these symptoms. Hidden foci of infection, especially in the jaws, prostate, and nose and throat, must be discovered. The patient must not be dieted and treated for allergy when any such pathology is causative.

EPILEPSY

Allergic epilepsy, whether associated with convulsions or with petit mal manifestations, has been reported by various allergists frequently enough to emphasize the importance of considering allergy as one possible cause in all so-called idiopathic cases. This is especially necessary in young children and adults in whom all neurological and other examinations have revealed no evident etiology. Food allergy has been incriminated in certain patients and inhalant allergies, both to animal emanations, miscellaneous allergens, and dusts, and also to pollens, have been proved responsible in a few individuals. The writer has studied about 30 patients with epilepsy with excellent results in a limited number. One patient had typical Jacksonian attacks starting in the small finger of the right hand. Egg allergy, not demonstrated by a skin reaction, was entirely causative. These experiences stress the importance of a thorough consideration of all possible allergic causes in these patients with idiopathic epilepsy. If relief is possible in even only 3 to 10 per cent of such cases, the routine allergic investigation is fully warranted. As in all patients suspected of allergy, the study must be conducted according to the methods outlined in this volume and the absolute coöperation of the patient is mandatory.

NEURAL ALLERGY

Localized allergy in different peripheral nerves may occur, especially from food allergy. The paresthesias and pareses, and even paralyses which develop in serum sickness, exemplify the possibility of other types of allergy affecting the spinal cord, the peripheral nerves and their membranes. Therefore, *neuralgia and peripheral pains which resist ordinary therapy may, in a few patients,* be due to food or other type of allergy. Neuralgic pains in the chest, arms, and shoulders which suggest possible angina pectoris may be due to food allergy. Adequate cardiac examination, of course, should rule out real pathology. Likewise, neuralgic pain in lower back, and legs, may be due to food allergy. Synovial membrane allergy, as discussed on page 136, also may be present. Patients with dizziness and some with *Ménière's syndrome* need to be studied from the allergic viewpoint, especially with food allergy as one possibility.

OCULAR ALLERGY

Conjunctival and scleral congestion, redness, watery or mucoid discharge with itching and light sensitiveness may or may not be associated with seasonal or perennial nasal allergy or bronchial asthma. *All of the various inhalants,* especially pollens, dusts, orris root, pyrethrum, karaya gum, kapok, cottonseed, and animal emanations, described in Chapter III, may be responsible. When such ocular allergy is severe and persistent, vernal catarrh may develop. The cobblestone changes in the conjunctiva are probably polypoid in nature. Lesions of the lids at times occur, simulating those of trachoma. Recently Bowen reported good results with the injection of oil antigens of causative pollens.

Food allergy may produce chronic conjunctival and scleral allergy. Such symptoms are usually non-seasonal. There is also photophobia and irritation of the eyes with mucoid discharge, but no severe itching when food allergy is the cause.

Corneal ulcers may result from recurrent food allergy and, at times, to drug inhalant and bacterial allergies. Eosinophiles may be present in the ocular mucus. The fact that corneal ulcers frequently occur in allergic patients speaks for the importance of an allergic etiology.

Drugs may produce ocular allergy. Thus, belladonna, mercury, zinc, quinine, chloral, cocaine, and other analgesics may be responsible. They may produce dermatitis on the eyelids or lesions of the eye and its conjunctivæ.

Iritis and uveitis often are due to bacterial allergy from some distant focus of infection.   Removal of the focus is necessary and careful hyposensitization with autogenous vaccines may be required.   It is likely that these lesions may also arise from *food or inhalant allergy* in a few individuals, although definite confirmation of this has not been possible.

Allergy apparently develops after cataract removal in some patients to the lens protein.   When a second cataract is removed, this lens allergy causes a severe ocular reaction in the operated eye due to the release of the lens allergen.   *Uveal pigment allergy* may also develop after a severe injury to the eye.   In two or three weeks after allergy has developed, an ophthalmic reaction may occur from such pigment allergy that may destroy sight and necessitate the removal of the eye.

Dermatitis of the lids or blepharitis associated with swelling, itching, oozing, crusting, or scaling of the skin of both lids may arise from food and especially from inhalant allergy.   When it occurs from early spring into the late fall, various pollens must be suspected.   Contact allergy may have to be considered.   When perennial dermatitis is present, food allergy and various inhalants encountered throughout the year should be considered.   Such blepharitis may be the beginning evidence of a spreading atopic or, less often, a contact dermatitis which involves the face, neck, upper chest and back, the flexures, and the extremities, as described previously in this chapter.

ALLERGIC ARTHROPATHIES

Allergy may develop in the synovial membranes of the joints and, at times, in the tendon sheaths.   Stiffness, swelling, soreness, and aching may result.   A few or many joints may be affected. Deformity rarely occurs, although some evidence indicates that with prolonged chronic involvements, it may arise.   The reaction may be intermittent or more or less persistent.   So-called *intermittent hydrarthrosis* of the larger joints probably is always due to allergy.   These rather sudden swellings with fluid formation in the joints, especially in the knee, may persist for one week or more with practically complete freedom between the attacks, or may gradually become chronic.   These arthropathies may be the only allergic manifestation, or may be accompanied by any of those discussed in this chapter.   *Food allergy is the most frequent cause.*   When the large joints are involved, the foods excluded from the routine elimination diets, especially wheat, milk, and eggs, must receive primary study. *Fruit allergy*, as discussed on page 124, must also be remembered, particularly when many of the small joints are affected. *Bacterial allergy and infrequently pollen allergy* may be responsible for a few of these synovial membrane reactions.

Bacterial allergy, particularly, may play a rôle in chronic arthritis of the atrophic or rheumatoid type and especially acute inflammatory rheumatism. Such allergy may arise from bacterial foci in teeth, tonsils, sinuses, pelvis, gall-bladder, appendix, rectum, prostate, and other regions of the body. It is possible that it might develop from the mucosal bacteria in the nose, throat, bronchi or gastro-intestinal tract. The fact that chronic arthritis can also be due to degenerative or hypertrophic changes, to trauma, to metabolic and nutritional disturbances and to neurogenic causes, must be remembered. These possibilities and the rôle of allergy in arthropathies have been more fully discussed in the writer's larger textbook on allergy.

UROGENITAL ALLERGY

The urogenital tissues may be the seat of localized allergy. They may be the main or the only shock tissues in the patient. Usually, other manifestations of allergy, however, are more pronounced. *Bladder allergy* most frequently occurs. Burning and frequent urination with cramping and urgency without urinary or cystoscopic findings indicate the possibility of allergy. Positive findings with such examinations, however, may occur along with bladder allergy. *The so-called Hunner's ulcers may be canker-like lesions in the bladder mucosa* and due to localized allergy. *Allergy may affect the kidney, pelvis, the ureter, the urethra,* causing congestion, edema, spasm, and even colic simulating that due to kidney or ureteral stone. Allergic inflammation, edema, or localized herpes or canker-like lesions may involve the external genitalia of man and woman. As with all symptoms suggestive of possible allergy, thorough physical examinations, laboratory tests, indicated cystoscopic and x-ray studies are imperative before allergy can receive definite consideration.

The uterus is probably susceptible to allergic reactivity as are other body tissues. Spasm in the musculature with edema of the mucosa could explain some dysmenorrhea. *Edema in the Fallopian tubes* has been described. *Vaginal congestion* and swelling from allergy at times occur. *Leucorrhea may be due to allergy* as is the mucus from the bronchial mucosa in bronchial asthma and the mucus from the colonic membrane in mucous colitis.

CARDIOVASCULAR ALLERGY

It has been suggested by certain students that *the primary seat of most atopic allergy may be in the vascular tissues* and that other tissues during the actual reaction are later affected. Since all atopic allergy is due to *blood-borne* ingestant, inhalant, injectant, or bacterial allergens, such vascular sensitization needs definite consideration. *Increased permeability with resultant transudation of fluid into the surrounding tissues is a most important result of allergy, the location depending on the area in which the greatest localized sensitization is present. Smooth muscle spasm in the walls of the blood-vessels* and even in the small islands of smooth muscle present on the walls of the capillaries (Rouget cells) may be due to allergy. The *contraction of the capillaries seen under a capillary microscope when tobacco smoke is inhaled* may be due to tobacco allergy causing such smooth muscle spasm.

Because of the possibilities of such vascular allergy, various vascular symptoms and lesions have been studied from the allergic viewpoint. Much evidence points to the probability that *thrombo-angiitis obliterans* may be due to ingestant or inhalant allergy, particularly to tobacco. The fact that eosinophilia is so marked in most patients with *periarteritis nodosa* and that the microscopic necroses around the arterial vessels in the body tissues usually are filled with eosinophiles have suggested an allergic etiology to many students. The possibility of generalized spasm throughout the arterial system due to allergy, as noted above, has suggested such a cause in some patients with *essential hypertension*. Some cases of *angina pectoris* might be due to vascular allergy in the cardiac tissues, as suggested in few articles in the literature. Localized vascular lesions characterizing *erythema nodosum* also necessitate a study of possible allergy in the etiology. Finally, *various cardiac irregularities*, especially paroxysmal tachycardia, seem to occur rather frequently in allergic patients and favorable results have been reported from the control of ingestant or inhalant allergies in such individuals. Changes in electrocardiographic tracings have disappeared in some patients when their allergies have been controlled. *As yet definite evidence has not been assembled that any of these manifestations are due to allergy. At present, it is justifiable to consider allergy as a possible cause in most of these conditions using the methods of study and treatment discussed in this volume.*

ALLERGY IN INFANT AND CHILDHOOD

Infants and children are subject to many allergic manifestations, especially when a definite positive family history of allergy is present. This is particularly true when marked allergy occurs in both sides of the family. Though many of these manifestations have been discussed in this chapter they deserve further emphasis.

Gastro-intestinal allergy is common in infancy. Much of the *colic, regurgitation, distention, diarrhea and at times constipation* of early months is due to this cause. The apparent disagreements and aversions for foods often result from allergy thereto. The various substitutes for milk when allergy to it exists have been discussed on page 199. *Pylorospasm* is at times due to food allergy. When pyloric hypertrophy is present, the rôle of allergy is questionable. *Canker sores* are usually due to food allergy, though, as noted on page 128, drug and at times bacterial allergy must be remembered. Later in childhood, recurrent or *cyclic vomiting* at times leading to acidosis is usually a forerunner of the sick headaches and allergic migraine of later years. (See page 132.)

Eczema occurs throughout infancy and childhood. Its identity with atopic dermatitis and its treatment have been discussed on page 118. Briefly, infantile eczema develops usually on the face and later on the flexures of the arms and legs, involving, at times, other areas of the body. Food allergy and occasionally inhalant allergy are the usual causes in infancy. As age increases, inhalant allergy becomes more important, though food allergy may be the complicating or sole cause throughout life.

It must be remembered that *excoriations and chafing in infants* require study of possible food allergies. *Pruritus ani* from allergic inflammation with consequent excoriation may arise from food allergy. Here allergy to an infection with monilia or possibly other fungi must be considered.

Hives are common in these years and are often vesicular. Such urticaria is usually due to fruit, egg and less often to other food allergies. The other causes of urticaria and *angioneurotic edema*, which are infrequent in infancy and childhood, have been outlined on page 122.

Contact allergy may occur at any age. Its causes have been noted on page 99. In early years it is not especially common. Allergy to fabrics, dyes, animal emanations, and vegetable resins, especially to those of poison oak and ivy is most important.

The *recurrent head cold and the intermittent or persistent nasal blocking*, congestion and sneezing, with or without watery or mucoid discharge must always suggest possible allergy. Such patients are devoid of the intoxication, fever and especially of the red, inflamed mucosa arising from an infectious cold. *Eosinophiles are often found* in the secretions and the pale, boggy mucosa is evident. These symptoms are more fully discussed in relation to allergy on page 116. The importance of pollens as a cause of nasal and ocular symptoms in the spring, summer and fall, and of animal emanations, of various miscellaneous allergens and of house and environmental dusts as causes of perennial symptoms is there noted. The necessity of considering food allergy, particularly when the symptoms are exaggerated from September to April, during which period food allergy is accentuated (see page 58), must be remembered.

Bronchial asthma or recurrent bronchitis may develop during later infancy, but usually at the end of the second year, especially when infantile eczema, if present, has decreased. As discussed on page 110, *food allergy* is the most common cause, especially when intermittent attacks are present. *Inhalant allergy* becomes more frequent as years advance and may be the sole cause or a complicating one along with food sensitizations. The allergic nature of *croup*, in most instances, must be appreciated.

The so-called *allergic toxemia*, the occurrence of *fever* without any evidence of infection or other causes, the *undernourishment* and impaired physical development, and especially the *anorexia* due to uncontrolled food and less often inhalant allergies, have already been described in this chapter. Most careful physical examination and laboratory tests must rule out all other possible pathology before allergy is given definite consideration. Tuberculin tests should be routine.

Both *petit and grand mal attacks of epilepsy and various epileptic equivalents* have been reported so often due to food and at times to inhalant and bacterial allergy that the possible rôle of allergy deserves thorough and adequate consideration in all so-called idiopathic cases. Careful neurological studies are important in such patients before allergy is given prolonged study. *Many children, moreover, are nervous, irritable, incorrigible, drowsy, or are unable to concentrate or study effectively* because of unrecognized or uncontrolled allergies. Susceptibility to nightmares, insomnia, phobias, bursts of temper, sullenness, or depression may result from chronic allergy. *Enuresis* at times will disappear when allergy is properly treated.

CHAPTER V

THE ELIMINATION DIETS*

Necessity of Detailed Menus.—Because of the necessity of remaining on the elimination diet, often for long periods of time in order to study adequately the possibilities of food allergy, *it is important that the foods be prescribed so that satisfying meals can be prepared and so that nutrition, above all else, is not damaged. By using the available knowledge of nutrition, these elimination diets can be arranged so that adequate nutrition is assured.* The writer's routine elimination diets contain carbohydrates, meats, vegetables, fruits, sugar, oil, and salt which permit the preparation of meals containing soup, salad, meat, vegetables, bread, jelly or jam, dessert, and a beverage as shown in printed menus on page 158.

Too often, when patients are only told to exclude positively reacting foods from the diet, satisfying meals are impossible and nutrition is endangered unless the physician painstakingly writes out a menu with foods allowed, and unless he assures himself that the patient's nutrition thereby is protected. Other disadvantages of the test-negative diet are discussed on page 14.

To obviate this danger with the elimination diets, detailed menus have been arranged and published previously and have been modified and extended in this volume. Even with such menus, however, it is important for the physician, and if possible for the patient, to determine the approximate amounts of protein, calories, vitamins, and minerals in the diet actually eaten, and to increase or supplement any which are below the normal requirements for the age and weight of the patient. (See page 206.) Such balancing of the diet has been discussed on page 146.

Time Necessary to Obtain Results With the Diets.—It is important to remember *that food allergy and other types of allergy which have existed for months and especially that which so often has existed for years, probably produce changes in the tissues which are persistent and, at times, irreversible in type.* Therefore, absolute freedom from the allergens to which these injured cells are sensitive, often for weeks and at times for months, should be assured in order to allow as much return to normal cellular structure and function as possible. The time necessary to restore

---

* The elimination diets are diagnostic tools for the study of possible food allergy, as are urinary tests for possible diabetes or nephritis or the Wassermann reaction for syphilis. Their use does not imply *a priori* that the physician has decided that the patient is suffering from food allergy.

cellular structure and function may be comparable to the time required for a bruise or wound to heal. Moreover, *it is possible that food and other allergens remain in the blood and body tissues for days, weeks, and possibly traces of them for months.* The speed of their elimination or destruction undoubtedly varies in different patients. Their persistence probably helps to explain the recurrence or continuation of symptoms in certain patients for several weeks after the allergenic foods have been completely removed from the diet. *These considerations, therefore, emphasize the importance of holding a patient to the prescribed elimination diet for at least two or three weeks and often for several months. Thus it is unfortunate that the idea has beeen written into the literature that food allergy can be excluded if the symptoms are not relieved by an elimination or test-negative diet in a few days.*

The time necessary to use elimination diets for the study of possible food allergy varies with the patient's problem. If daily or bi-weekly symptoms disappear during the first two weeks of dieting and similar relief has not occurred for months before, then it can be assumed that the foods productive of allergy in the patient are absent from the diet. Foods, thereafter, can gradually be added as suggested on page 156.

When symptoms recur every two to four weeks, relief will have to be present for two or three months before adequate evidence is obtained that the allergenic foods have been removed. In such cases as stressed elsewhere in this book, inhalant, bacterial, and contactant allergics must receive constant attention in many patients while symptoms continue and while the possibilities of food allergy are being studied. *Thus, the time that the initial elimination diet should be used varies with the frequency with which the patient's symptoms have recurred. When they only recur for a day or so every two to six months*, prolonged diet trial is not justifiable unless serious symptoms such as asthma or epilepsy warrant prolonged study with elimination diets. If the symptoms are very suggestive of food allergy and are severe and invaliding, then various elimination diets, as suggested on page 134, may be justified if necessary over a period of three to six months before the possible control of the symptoms by the elimination of allergenic foods is given up. *Such prolonged diet manipulation, of course, demands protection of nutrition and weight as stressed on page* 146. After symptoms are relieved, additional foods must be added— one or two every week—as recommended on page 145. The fact that allergenic reactions from such foods may appear in a few hours or only after two or three weeks of inclusion in the diet, again must be recalled. *This, of necessity, makes the final determination of the degree and time of reactivity of such foods a long procedure in certain patients, and demands absolute coöperation and much persistence and fortitude in patient and in physician alike.* The relief of chronic asthma, nasal allergy, eczema, longstanding gastro-intestinal symptoms, recurrent headache, migraine, or other allergic symptoms often present for years, at times since childhood, fully justifies prolonged diet manipulation. At all times, other possible influences on the symptoms such as climate, seasons, nervousness, and the relief of other diseased states than allergy must be in mind in evaluating the possible rôle of food allergy. The only requirement with such dieting, it must be stressed over and over again, is that nutritional requirements be adequately met by the diets prescribed. If this is not possible according to the directions on page 146, elimination diets should be discontinued.

It must be emphasized that *the patient suspected of or afflicted with allergy must be studied not only with the possibility of food allergy in mind, but also with the realization that all types of inhalant, bacterial, or contactant allergies may be present.* The emphasis on food allergy in this and other chapters does not mean that the writer would ignore in the slightest degree other types of sensitization.

THE PERSISTENCE OF FOOD ALLERGY

Food sensitizations tend to diminish or disappear as the foods are eliminated from the diet. At times, their elimination for one or two months reduces the allergic tissue reactivity so that they can be eaten without the previous symptomatology. At times, such foods must be omitted entirely from the diet for six to twelve months or for several years before tolerance returns. Vaughan concludes that on the average a food must be excluded for four and one-half years before it can be eaten without obvious allergic symptoms. Too often food allergy persists for many years even though causative foods are excluded from the diet. In childhood there is a tendency to a gradual disappearance of food sensitizations, and the same holds true during the late forties and fifties. *The symptoms due to allergy may gradually diminish, but the potential allergy usually persists and, in a short time or even years later, other allergic symptoms may develop from the same foods.* Thus, infantile eczema may disappear and asthma may arise in the second or third year; gastro-intestinal allergy in childhood may be supplanted by recurrent sick headaches or migraine in adolescence.

The diminution of food allergy by hyposensitization with gradually increasing doses of the allergens of the causative foods has failed except in a rare patient. Patients are so sensitive to such food allergens in many instances that an infinitesimal dose such as 0.10 cc. of a 1 to 1,000,000 dilution of the allergen will reproduce the symptoms. At times gradually increasing doses apparently are tolerated and finally foods can be taken without symptoms. In such cases it is always possible that the foods in question never caused actual allergy. The attempt to increase tolerance to definitely allergenic foods by increasing doses of such foods by mouth has failed in the hands of most allergists. The good results which apparently arise are often with foods which mistakenly have been adjudged allergic by the patient or physician.

Thus, the way by which food allergy can best be decreased is by the elimination of the food from the diet. The more complete this is, the more hope there should be that tolerance will be established. This necessity of eliminating allergenic foods for varying periods of time, too often for many years, requires absolute assurance of the physician and patient that the elimination diet necessary for the relief of the patient's symptoms is balanced adequately to protect nutrition and weight, as discussed on page 146.

THE ELIMINATION DIETS (Second Revision)

When these diets were first published in 1928, five diets were proposed, four containing one or more cereal grains and the fifth containing milk. In 1933, these diets were revised so that the first two contained one or more cereal grains, the third was cereal-free, depending on tapioca, potato, and the legumes for its starches. The fourth contained milk.

For several years, continued experience has indicated a few helpful changes in the revised elimination diets. Cottonseed oil and shortenings have been excluded. The frequency of allergy to cottonseed was noted in 1933 and since then sesame oil and sesame shortening have been substituted, since allergy thereto is extremely rare. Olive oil is still included, though it should be excluded when a positive reaction to olive allergen and even to olive pollen exists. The adulteration of certain commercial olive oils with other edible oils necessitates the assurance of unquestioned purity of the chosen olive oil. Finally, all legumes have been excluded from Diets 1 and 2.

Cereal-free Elimination Diet.— *During the last few years, the cereal-free elimination diet has been used in preference to the diets* *containing cereal grains since group sensitizations to two or more cereal grains often exists, especially if wheat allergy is present.* Moreover, the initial cereal-free diet has included all of the meats, vegetables, and fruits in the routine elimination Diets 1, 2, and 3, plus soy, lima, potato, and tapioca for carbohydrates. This has given a wider variety of foods to which allergy infrequently exists and more acceptable menus have been possible. As published in 1937, moreover, when the initial diet has contained rice, corn, or rye, **a combination menu of Diets 1 and 2** has been used. *Thus, two elimination diets are now being used for the initial study af the patients suspected of food allergy.* The cereal-free 1, 2, and 3 diet is preferred. When intolerance for legumes, however, is indicated by history, skin testing, or actual distress after eating them, then Diets 1 and 2 in combination are used. For selected patients, Diets 1, 2, and 3 are still individually available and the menus are published in this book for their possible use.

The initial diet should also be modified as follows: If there is a definite history of aversion or intolerance, or if a definite positive skin reaction by the scratch test is present to any foods, such foods should be suspected of causing allergy and they should be eliminated. Other foods of similar caloric, vitamin, and protein content may be added if the deletion of the former foods impairs the patient's menus.

If relief occurs after the cereal-free 1, 2, and 3 diet has been used for an adequate period as discussed on page 141, then rice and corn and later rye may be added. So that the patient may appreciate the ways in which these cereals may be added, possibilities are detailed on pages 201. If, on the other hand, the cereal containing Diets 1 and 2 have been initially used and have given relief, then if no apparent intolerance to legumes exists, they may be added, including peas, string beans, lima and soy beans, according to the suggestions detailed in the menus on page 158.

As relief continues, the following foods, one or two at a time, may be added at one to two week intervals. The varying degree and possible time of reactions from such added foods as discussed on page 56, must be remembered. *The influence of seasons and of proximity to the ocean must be kept in mind.* (See page 58.) Cherries, figs, avocado, cranberry, rhubarb, celery, egg plant, cauliflower, cabbage, sprouts, broccoli, banana, apple, orange, melons, ham, pork, fin and shell fish, rabbit, duck, and game birds may be tried. Other unusual foods such as taro, papaya and other tropical foods when available may be tested individually. The time for the trial of egg, milk and its products, and wheat depends on the

10

patient's history and the physician. If definite evidence of allergy to any of these common foods exists, it may be unwise to add such to the diet until the symptoms have been absent for months, during which time tolerance may have been restored. Since the food allergens and the tissue reactions may persist in the body for weeks or even longer, as noted on page 141, the addition of a food which has been a definite cause of allergy in the past may be unwise too soon after relief has arisen.

The addition of various beverages needs discussion. In the initial diet, because of the frequency of allergy to coffee, it should be excluded. It may be tried if desired soon after definite relief has occurred. The fact that egg is often added to clear coffee and that chicory, to which occasional allergy is present, is also contained in some grinds, must be remembered. Allergy to tea is less frequent. However, in the initial diet it is best excluded. It may be added as symptomatic relief becomes definite. The autonomic nervous system of many allergic patients is very sensitive and the elimination of coffee and tea is also beneficial because of their caffein content.

In the initial diet, *the specified fruit and tomato juices* are included. Too large amounts, however, may cause digestive disturbances and decreased appetite. The possible inclusion of corn glucose in certain canned juices and of spices in some tomato juice must be considered, especially if such foods have not been added to the diet. The use of soy bean substitutes for milk in the presence of cow's milk allergy will be discussed on page 199. A moderately thick puree of split peas, salted, and flavored with a little bacon or ham shank and served hot or cold, makes a fair substitute for milk. This may be given to young children as a drink or a soup or may be acceptable to older children and even adults. Canned pea soups, because of the varying content of other foods and spices, should not be taken. Plain puree of peas, of course, is allowable. Puree of soy bean (see page 253) however, is more desirable since its protein contains essential amino acids present in milk and not found in other legumes. (See page 82.)

The graphic recording of the foods first ordered for the patient with subsequent additions and subtractions is easily accomplished with the form as printed on page 217.

MAINTENANCE OF NUTRITION

As stressed throughout this book, *nutrition must be maintained at all times when elimination diets are being given.* While egg and milk products are excluded, *adequate protein* intake requires the eating of a good amount of the specified meat at least twice a day. Bacon may also be taken, although its protein content varies. Legumes, when emphasized in the diet, add considerably to the protein intake. *The approximate vitamin content of the foods in the diet* can be estimated by referring to published tables. (See page 203.) If the amount of any of the vitamins is deficient, then additional A, B, C, D, and E should be given. If A is necessary, Caritol, preferably in sesame oil or in corn oil if corn is on the diet, may be given. Until fish is prescribed, cod-liver or other fish oils should not be ordered. Thiamin and the B complex may be given if the diet is low in these vitamins. Preparations containing wheat germ or rice polishings should not be used until these foods are added to the diet. Cevitamic acid in from 50 to 100 mg. amounts should be taken if allergy to citrus fruits exists. It must be remembered, however, that many of the vegetables and other fruits, as shown in published tables, contain considerable amounts of vitamin C. The regular elimination diets are deficient in vitamin D. Thus, if sun exposure or sun lamp is not available, Viosterol, preferably in sesame oil or Drisdol should be given. If fish has been added, then the vitamin D rich fish oils or their concentrates may be used.

The elimination of milk usually results in a deficiency of calcium in the diet. Sherman recommends that 1 gram of available calcium be taken in the diet daily. Milk contains about 1.2 grams to each quart. For each menu of the elimination diets in this Chapter of this book, the amount of calcium has been estimated. The additional amount of calcium to meet the daily requirement of 1 gram should be taken in one of the calcium salts. Calcium carbonate is the cheapest source and 40 per cent of its weight is available calcium. One teaspoonful* weighs about 2.2 grams and thus contains 0.88 grams of available calcium. Dicalcium phosphate contains 24 per cent calcium. One teaspoonful weighs 3.5 grams and contains 0.8 gram of calcium and 0.6 gram of phosphorus. Because of its phosphorus content, it is indicated especially in infancy when milk and meat free diets are prescribed. Calcium gluconate is the most soluble salt but only contains 9 per cent available calcium. One teaspoonful weighs 2 grams and thus only contains 0.18 gram of calcium.

When anemia is present, additional iron may be required as determined by the physician's blood count. Allergy to all iron preparations at times occurs.

---

* One teaspoonful is the amount in a level, moderately packed standard measuring teaspoon.

With diet tables, the approximate amounts of protein, carbohydrate, fat, calories, calcium, phosphorus, and iron have been
figured for the menus specified for Diets 1 and 2 and Cereal-free
diets. The approximate amounts of Vitamins A, B, C, D and G
should be determined by the use of published values. (See page
203.) Additional calcium and vitamins must be taken whenever
the requirements are not satisfied by the actual ingested foods.
The nutritional requirements of these various elements in the
diet and the caloric requirements for various ages are tabulated
on page 206.

MAINTENANCE AND INCREASE OF WEIGHT

When the diet contains the number of calories required for ths
patient's age and satisfies the nutritional requirements, as discussed above, then weight should increase or be maintained according to the age. *If loss of weight arises, more of the calorie carrying
foods, namely the carbohydrates, sugars, and fats in the diet should
be taken. Specific directions for such increase of these various foods
are detailed on page 207.* If weight loss occurs in spite of such extra
intake of food, the physician must be certain that some disease
other than allergy is not present. *The general health of the patient,
as well as his allergic problem, must always be under control.* At
times, weight loss is due to impaired digestive function and is
stopped when required dilute hydrochloric acid, pepsin, or pancreatic ferments are given. As the diet is continued, weight must
be recorded every two or three days so that undue loss of weight
can be forestalled.

When gradual increase in weight and height is necessary, as in
children, such results may not occur for several weeks or a few
months after the diet has been started even though adequate
calories are taken. Weight increase occurs at definite intervals
in children and remains stationary at other periods.

*The fact that uncontrolled allergy, especially to foods, often accounts
for lack of appetite and leads to undernutrition,* as noted on page
140, must be remembered. Children who have been spoon fed all
their lives often develop good or ravenous appetites when the
allergenic foods are eliminated.

NECESSITY OF ABSOLUTE ACCURACY IN DIETING

*The patient must not eat or taste a trace of food not prescribed in
his elimination diet. It is only when the physician is certain that
this is being done that he can make correct deductions regarding the*

effect of the diet.   Above all else, the patient must not deceive himself and his physician during trial dieting by making conscious or unconscious mistakes, large or small, in his food intake.   To be certain that the necessary strictness in dieting is understood, the physician should interview or communicate with the patient at frequent intervals, at first every week or two.   He should be sure that *the patient is not tasting forbidden foods, that foods are being cooked in clean utensils and served in clean dishes, that spices and condiments are not being used unless specifically ordered, that the specified oils and shortenings are being employed, that cooks in home, restaurant, or hotel are not making any of these mistakes and are not stirring or serving food with unwashed spoons or knives* that have just been used in forbidden foods such as milk, soup, or custard, if they are excluded.   As stressed on page 155, it must be assured that *bakery products are being made according to recipes furnished by the physician* with specified flours, shortenings, sugars, and flavors in the home or *by bakers whose honesty is unquestioned.* So-called soy, lima, rice, or potato bread as ordinarily baked usually contains wheat or gluten flours and often milk, egg, or cottonseed shortening.   It is impossible to make a yeast-raised bread of the above flours which is at all light without the addition of wheat or gluten flours.   Thus, to be sure about such bakery products, it is usually necessary to be certain that the soy, lima, or other flour first of all is pure and unadulterated.   Then the physician or patient should watch the actual making of the bread, cake, or cookie to be sure that only these flours and other ingredients specified in the recipes and no trace of any other food are used in the process.   The baking of the product should be watched even until taken from the oven.   He will then know the quality and texture which can be obtained when honest preparation occurs. Similar products from that baker can probably be depended upon in the future.

The use of canned or prepared mixtures of foods such as soups, preserves, sauces, mayonnaise, catsups, sausages, and many others *is forbidden.*   Even though the ingredients are printed on the container or wrapper according to the new pure food law, it cannot be assured that all the ingredients have been included or that they, temporarily, have not been changed.   *Soups,* if used, should only be eaten in the patient's home where their contents can be accurately determined.   Whether or not the use of corn glucose or other forbidden sugar in *jellies or preserves* will cause allergy in a corn sensitive individual is not certain, but for accuracy, such sugars should be excluded until actually added to the diet by the physician. *Similar critical analysis of all other foods and their preparation is necessary.*

MEALS AWAY FROM HOME OR IN HOTELS OR RESTAURANTS

Eating away from home in friends' houses, restaurants, hotels, or on trains always is difficult for accurate dieting. Since a taste of a forbidden food, even once a week, may prevent disappearance of allergic symptoms, it is most important during the period of diet trial to forego eating a suspected food or even an entire meal if there is any question about the ingredients of the foods therein. One can always eat in an hour or two afterward and fasting for several hours will do no harm in the majority of cases. *The taste or small amount of a food that "will do no harm" may delay good results for one to three weeks as noted on page 141. Suggested menus for the cereal and cereal-free elimination diets obtainable away from home are printed on pages 177–180.* If eating in restaurants, hotels, or boarding houses is constantly necessary, usually a *coöperative and understanding cook* can be found who will prepare the meals accurately if specific menus and recipes are provided by the patient.

In brief, a patient can safely take the following foods: Plain salad containing the vegetables on the diet. For a salad dressing, lemon or vinegar, if allowed, with salt may be added. Only a specified oil should be used. If necessary, a small bottle of sesame or pure olive or other allowed oil may be carried to the meal. Plain meat such as chops, steak, cold or hot roast beef or lamb may be obtained practically anywhere. Such should be broiled or fried in its own fat. No butter or other fat or pepper should be used. Roast meats should be served plain with no gravies or sauces, since away from home they invariably contain butter, flour, spices or flavors of varying types. Baked or boiled potatoes, white or sweet, served in their jackets can always be obtained. If necessary, the patient can wait in the restaurant while such are being cooked. Fried, mashed, or scalloped potatoes are forbidden unless the foods used in their preparation such as milk are allowed by the physician. Then plain vegetables on the diet may be eaten and canned fruit or possibly fresh fruit on the diet may be ordered. Such a meal can be obtained at practically any hotel, restaurant, or in the home of an understanding and coöperative friend, if the patient orders specifically and insists on accuracy of preparation. No bread or bakery products served away from home should be tasted. If Ry-Krisp has been added, it may be eaten. No butter, unless already added to the diet, should be eaten. The patient may carry a few slices of bread or cookies made at home or by the entrusted baker (see page 149) in his pocket to use at meals away from home. On trips lasting for days or weeks, such bakery products can be mailed at proper intervals. More detailed menus for meals away from home are presented on pages 177–180.

During the period of diet trial such meticulous care is most necessary if dependable conclusions regarding the effect of the diet in question are to be drawn. With a similar attitude and care, other elimination diets can usually be obtained away from home. It must be emphasized, however, *if weight maintenance is a problem, that the inclusion of adequate calories in the meals according to suggestions on page 207, is imperative. Nutrition, as emphasized on page 146, must also be maintained. If undesirable weight loss or nutritional impairment occurs, then the elimination diet must be stopped until a readjustment of dieting will assure prevention of such undesirable results.*

Most patients must be told on several occasions and at times, repeatedly, for months or even years, that strict adherence to the diet is necessary if the symptoms arising from specific food allergies are to be eliminated. Patients and especially their associates will argue that *"a little will do no harm"* or that a certain recipe contains no butter, milk, egg, wheat, or other food in question; but, unfortunately, it is such occasional and often small amounts of forbidden foods that keep the food allergy active and prevent the symptomatic relief which would otherwise be possible. *Such small amounts of food, moreover, can do no possible good except transient gratification of taste and relaxation from the necessary will power to maintain the strict diet.* The few calories and the other nutritional elements in such forbidden foods are not worthy of consideration. Thus, contrary to the usual statement, "this small amount" of a bread or dessert or cookie will do great harm and is often responsible for the failure to obtain the relief so important for the patient's welfare.

SUPPLEMENTAL ELIMINATION DIETS

When the regular Diets 1, 2, or 3 fail to relieve symptoms, then the supplemental elimination diets may be necessary if definite indications of food allergy exist, or such diets may be used initially if sensitizations to many different foods or to nearly all members of one or more groups of foods such as cereals, fruits, vegetables, or meats are indicated by history or possibly by skin reactions. At times, allergy to biologically related vegetables or fruits such as legumes, citrus or pit fruits exists or may be suspected.

Thus in the unsolved case of possible food allergy, all foods must be suspected and minimal trial diets may be arranged containing the following foods:

1. A choice of one or two of the following carbohydrates: rice corn, tapioca, sago, taro, sweet or white potato.

2. A choice of one or two of the following protein rich foods: lamb, beef, chicken, soy bean.

3. A choice of two or three of the following vegetables: spinach, carrot, beet, artichoke, asparagus, pea, string bean, tomato.

4. A choice of one or two of the following fruits: lemon, grapefruit, pear, peach, apricot, pineapple.

5. Mazola (corn), olive or sesame oil, white sugar, maple syrup, corn glucose.

If sensitization to whole or partial groups of foods such as all ruits, rarely to all vegetables, citrus or pit fruits, legumes or other related foods is at all likely, then such groups should be excluded, provided that the prescribed diet and its carefully prepared menus meet metabolic and caloric requirements. Such menus for a fruit-free elimination diet are found on pages 171 to 175 and 181. Other similar menus for elimination diets minus legumes and cereals, meats or all vegetables and fruits may be prepared. *The choice of the supplemental diet depends on the patient's history of food dislikes or disagreements, on actual clinical reactions to foods evident from diet trial and on definite skin reactions to food allergens. The fallibility of the skin reactions to foods,* especially by the intradermal test, as discussed on page 13, however, must be kept in mind. Such diets, moreover, must contain the required amount of protein and as many vitamins as possible with the foods prescribed. The patient's vitamin and mineral requirements must be satisfied, if necessary, with extra vitamins as stressed on page 146. Unless weight reduction is desired, *these supplemental diets should be used only by patients who coöperate by eating sufficient calories of the specified foods to maintain weight. In childhood, proper weight increase should occur.*

MODIFICATION OF ELIMINATION DIETS IN THE PRESENCE OF OTHER DISEASES*

When patients have a marked gastro-intestinal syndrome such as "colitis" or peptic ulcer, the prescribed elimination diet can be

---

* For reduction elimination diets for patients suspected of allergy see page 187.

prepared in a *smooth, non-irritating form*. This can be effected by the pureeing or straining of all fruits and vegetables and the cooking of nearly all foods. Meats should be finely minced and carefully cooked with a minimum of grease. As the gastro-intestinal symptoms improve, the smooth diet can gradually be supplanted by the ordinary elimination diet and uncooked foods can gradually be added according to the patient's tolerance and relief of his symptoms. As noted on page 129, the increasing evidence indicates that certain cases of *ulcerative colitis* are due to food allergy and that a similar cause is responsible for many so-called *irritable or unstable colons*. In such cases, the smooth, non-irritating elimination diets, as here described, are indicated for diagnostic study of such possible allergy.

Food allergy rather frequently exists in the diabetic patient. When obvious sensitizations exist, those foods can be excluded, other similar foods being substituted so that no nutritional damage occurs. When food allergy is suspected as a possible cause of bronchial asthma, eczema, gastro-intestinal symptoms or sick headaches in a diabetic, then the diabetic diet must be chosen from the foods in the elimination diet selected for purposes of diagnostic study of such possible food allergy. *A typical diet of this type is detailed on page 195.* Other similar diets according to the patient's diabetic tolerance and his possible or definite food allergies can be arranged. The writer has studied several diabetics, especially children, who have had recurrent acidosis and threatened coma due to cyclic vomiting. As noted on page 132, evidence stresses the frequency with which this vomiting is due to food allergy, being a forerunner of sick headaches or recurrent migraine of later life. Other diabetics with gastro-intestinal symptoms, dermatitis, or asthma have been relieved by the exclusion from their diabetic diets of various foods found by diet trial to be responsible for their allergies. To prevent such recurrent vomiting, acidosis, and possible coma in these diabetics, the indicated elimination diet often has to be continued according to the patient's carbohydrate tolerance for several months or possibly years.

Gout and food allergy occasionally have been associated in the writer's patients and the elimination diet which controls the food allergy must also exclude those foods which are high in purins. Recently, a patient had painful swellings in feet, ankles, wrists, and a few other joints, which were not only due to synovial membrane allergy, but also to gout. Some students have suggested that gout is due to food allergy, but the experience of many others, including the writer, has not substantiated this idea.

The following elimination diets, as stated on page 144, have been slightly modified compared with those published in 1937. Cottonseed and olive oils because of varying allergy to them, have been omitted. Legumes have been included only in Diet 3, and a few other changes in vegetables have been made.

Elimination Diets (Rowe)

Diet 1	Diet 2	Diet 3	Diet 4
Rice	Corn	Tapioca	Milk*
Tapioca	Rye	White potato	Tapioca
Rice biscuit	Corn pone	Breads made of any	
Rice bread	Corn-rye muffin	combination of	
	Rye bread	soy, lima and	
	Ry-Krisp	potato flours and	
		tapioca	
Lettuce	Beets	Tomato	
Chard	Squash	Carrot	
Spinach	Asparagus	Lima beans	
Carrot	Artichoke	String beans	
Sweet potato or yam		Peas	
Lamb	Chicken	Beef	
	Bacon	Bacon	
Lemon	Pineapple	Lemon	
Grapefruit	Peach	Grapefruit	
Pears	Apricot	Peach	
	Prune	Apricot	
Cane sugar	Cane or beet sugar	Cane sugar	
Sesame oil	Mazola oil	Sesame oil	
Sesame spread	Sesame oil	Soy bean oil	
Salt	Sesame Spread	Sesame Spread	
Gelatin, plain or fla-	Salt	Gelatin, plain or fla-	
vored with lime	Gelatin, plain or fla-	vored with lime	
or lemon	vored with pine-	or lemon	
Maple syrup or	apple	Salt	
syrup made with	Karo corn syrup	Maple syrup or	
cane sugar fla-	White vinegar	syrup made with	
vored with maple	Royal baking pow-	cane sugar fla-	
Royal baking pow-	der	vored with maple	
der	Baking soda	Royal baking pow-	
Baking soda	Cream of tartar	der	
Cream of tartar	Vanilla extract	Baking soda	
Vanilla extract		Cream of tartar	
Lemon extract		Vanilla extract	
		Lemon extract	

*Milk should be taken up to two or three quarts a day. Plain cottage cheese and cream may be used. Tapioca cooked with milk and milk sugar may be taken.

USE OF ELIMINATION DIETS

(Important to Read and Follow)

Since skin tests with food allergens often are negative to allergenic foods or give false or positive reactions not associated with clinical allergy, the elimination diets are usually indicated for the study of the suspected food allergy. In some patients, test-negative diets excluding skin reacting foods control symptoms. (See page 14.)

1. Foods productive of possible allergy as suggested by history or skin reactions may be omitted and other similar foods substituted. (See page 145.)

2. No drop or trace of any food not ordered or included in the diet can be taken. Clean utensils and dishes free from traces of forbidden foods must be used. Spoons and knives must not be used unless washed free of all excluded foods such as milk, egg, wheat, etc. Tasting of any food off the diet is not allowed.

3. To increase caloric intake, 1 to $1\frac{1}{2}$ ounces of prescribed oil should be served in a pitcher with each meal, to be used on salads and vegetables as tolerated: the remainder may be taken between meals if weight increase is important. Plenty of the prescribed butter substitute, sugar, syrup, jam, jelly, potatoes, bread, peas, beans, tapioca cooked as above, with meals and between meals will increase calories. Frequent weighing on the same scale will indicate adequacy of caloric intake. (See page 146.) Prescribed meats must be taken twice daily to assure adequate protein and essential amino-acid intake. They must be cooked in their own fats or with prescribed oils or fats with salt but with no pepper, condiments, or garnishes. Bacon for breakfast is to be taken if tolerated. Gravies must be made with meat juices, salted, and thickened with prescribed flours, but with no condiments, onion, etc. Bakery products must be made by recipes in this volume by honest bakers or at home.

4. Approximate vitamin content of the daily diet should be determined by use of published tables. Vitamin A as Caritol and Vitamin D as Viosterol should be ordered in sesame or other oil allowed in the diet. Drisdol may also be used to supply D. Fish oils are contraindicated until fish is added to the diet. Vitamin B^1 should be given as Thiamin. B complex capsules containing Thiamin and the other synthetic B vitamins may be used.

Calcium gluconate—2 teaspoonfuls twice daily, dicalcium phosphate—1 teaspoonful daily, or calcium carbonate—1 teaspoonful, stirred in water, once a day on an empty stomach will assure calcium balance.

5. Sesame oil (Globe A-1 or other reliable brands) is preferred. Pure soy bean oil may be used. Olive oil is often adulterated, even when labeled pure. Allergy to olive at times occurs. Cottonseed allergy is so frequent that cottonseed products are not used in initial diets. Sesame Spread is made of hydrogenated Sesame Oil, salted to taste, with artificial color and butter flavor. Its use is optional.

6. The diet should be accurately taken for two or more weeks. (See page 141.) As definite relief of former symptoms occurs which is longer than former periods of relief, then additional foods in the other elimination diets can be added, one every five to seven days, their effects being carefully ascertained. (See page 145.) Detailed directions for addition of rice and corn to the cereal free diet are on page 201. Thereafter, other vegetables, fruits, meats, fowl, fish, spices, and nuts may gradually be added. In one to three months, milk, egg and wheat may be tried separately, one of them every two weeks. If the patient is allergic to any food, symptoms may occur immediately or in days or even weeks according to the patient's tolerance. Such food should be eliminated.

7. Hyposensitization by elimination of a food may require weeks, months or years. With the above precautions, caloric and metabolic requirements are assured with continued dieting.

8. The diagnostic control and treatment of inhalant, bacterial and contactant allergies which may accompany food sensitizations are most important and not infrequently are necessary for satisfactory control of a food allergy. The physician must supervise the accurate following of the elimination diet by frequent conferences or letters. Proper weight and nutrition must be maintained.

MENUS FOR THE ELIMINATION DIETS

Patients who have actual or possible allergy to foods must be told definitely what they can eat and must be provided with detailed menus so that adequate and satisfying meals can be prepared or procured, if necessary, away from home. If on the contrary they are only told to exclude certain foods, and no menus are provided, their diet trial in nearly every case will be filled with errors and, from a diagnostic standpoint, will become worthless.

Thus, as years have passed, I have provided my patients with increasingly more explicit menus and directions about the preparation of their meals. The patient is warned to eat only those foods included in his diet and to be certain at all times that a trace of a forbidden food is not eaten until such has been allowed by the physician. He is told to refuse any suspected food, remembering that a slight mistake might invalidate diet trial for a week or more. Missing the whole or part of a meal is never serious since proper food can be obtained within an hour or two. It is only with such careful analysis of his meals that the patient can do justice to the study of food allergy as a possible cause of his symptoms.

The various menus which follow have been prepared in more detail and with more practical suggestions than in my former publications. *For the routine patient, the Cereal-free Diet 1, 2 and 3 as noted on page 144 is usually preferred.* The combined menu for Diets 1 and 2 is also commonly used, especially if intolerance or allergy to legumes is present. Then, menus follow for these diets minus all fruits, which menus are of special use in urticaria, bladder allergy and other conditions where fruit allergy is suspected. Menus for both diets to be taken away from home, in hotels, restaurants or in friends' homes are detailed. Menus for Infants and Young Children have been arranged. Menus for Diets 1, 2 and 3 separately are included. Then various supplemental elimination diets are proposed.

All of these various menus may have to be changed by eliminations or substitutions according to definite skin reactions or history of food disagreements or dislikes as discussed on page 145. When individualized menus are necessary, the patient must be provided with detailed menus similar to those that follow so that no question can arise in his mind about the prescribed foods and the various ways in which they can be taken in order to maintain proper weight and nutrition. The amounts of the various foods taken by the patient must vary according to his caloric requirements as indicated in the Table on page 206.

As stressed throughout the book, elimination diets should never be prescribed unless proper nutrition and adequate weight maintenance are assured by the menu given the patient by the physician.

Cereal–free Elimination Diets 1, 2 and 3 (Rowe)
Foods Allowed

Tapioca	Carrots	Cane or beet sugar
White potato	Beets	Salt
Sweet potato or yam	Artichoke	Sesame oil
Lima bean potato bread	Tomato	Soy bean oil
Soy bean lima bean bread	Squash	Sesame Spread
	Asparagus	Gelatin, plain
Soy bean potato tapioca bread	Peas	Lime, lemon or pineapple flavored gelatin
	String beans	
	Lima beans	
Lamb		Maple syrup or syrup made with cane sugar
Beef		
Chicken (no hens)	Lemon	flavored with maple
Bacon	Grapefruit	White vinegar
	Pears	Vanilla extract
	Pineapple	Lemon extract
Lettuce	Peaches	Royal baking powder
Spinach	Apricots	Baking soda
Chard	Prunes	Cream of tartar

Suggested Menu
BREAKFAST

Beverage: Approximate Amounts

   (a) Fresh or canned grapefruit juice served with sugar.   4 to 6 oz.

   (b) Pineapple, apricot, peach, or prune juice, served singly
       or mixed with grapefruit juice.

   (c) Tomato juice (canned and unspiced).   5 to 8 oz.

Cereal Substitute:

   (a) Tapioca cooked with water or fruit juice and puréed   ½ cup
       apricots, peaches, prunes, or pineapple, served hot
       with juice of the fruit if desired.(1)

   (b) Tapioca cooked in water, sweetened with sugar and   ½ cup
       flavored with lemon juice and grated lemon rind, or
       cooked with caramelized sugar, brown sugar, or
       maple syrup.(2)

Meat:

   (a) Bacon   4 slices

   (b) Lamb chops, patties or tongue (unspiced).(3)   2 med. pats

   (c) Beefsteak, beef patties or tongue (unspiced).   2 med. pats

   (d) Calves, beef or lamb liver and bacon.   2 slices

*Bread:**

   (a) Lima bean-potato bread, soy bean-lima bean bread, or   2 slices
       soy bean-potato-tapioca bread, toasted.(4)

   (b) Lima bean-potato, soy bean-lima bean, or soy bean-   2 muffins
       potato-tapioca muffins.(5)

   (c) Pancakes or waffles made of soy, lima and potato   4 medium
       flours, served with Sesame Spread and maple syrup.
       (6)

* Name and address of supervised and trusted baker must be given by the physician.

Butter Substitute:

    Sesame Spread; salted, hydrogenated sesame oil or   1 Tbsp.
    bacon grease.

Jams or Preserves:

    (*a*) Jams made of pears, pineapple, peaches, apricots and   2 tsp.
    prunes, singly or in combination.(7)

    (*b*) Lemon, grapefruit or carrot marmalade.(8)

    (*c*) Tomato preserves flavored with lemon.(9)

    (*d*) Pear butter.(10b)

Fruit:

    (*a*) Fresh or canned grapefruit   ½ grapefruit

    (*b*) Fresh, cooked, or canned pears, pineapple, peaches or   1 peach or
    apricots. Fresh peeled pears, peaches and apricots   equivalent
    may be eaten raw if allowed by the physician.

    (*c*) Cooked dried prunes. Lemon juice and sugar may be   4 prunes
    added as desired. Do not use dried apricots or
    peaches.

This menu contains approximately 770 calories.

LUNCH OR DINNER

Soup:

    (*a*) Broth made of lamb, beef, or chicken (no hens) served   1 cup
    clear with tapioca or cooked with vegetables as pre-
    viously listed. (No pepper or spices, no canned
    soups and no soups away from home.)

    (*b*) Lima bean or split pea soup, plain, salted, flavored   1 cup
    with bacon.(11) (No milk, butter, or any other food
    to be added.)

Salad:

    Any combination of vegetables or fruits listed in this diet,   ½ cup veg.
    dressing only of Sesame oil, white vinegar or lemon juice,   or fruit
    salt and sugar.(12) (Variations: [1] Lime or lemon flav-   1 Tbsp. oil
    ored gelatin with grated raw carrots or crushed pineapple.
    [2] Cooked sliced beets pickled in white vinegar, season
    with salt and sugar. [3] Cut young tender carrots into
    long thin strips and place in iced salted water for one-
    half hour. Use as an appetizer or as a garnish for salads.)

Meat:

    (*a*) Lamb and beef—chops, steak, tongue or liver, ground   Av. liberal
    plain meat, roast (hot or cold) cooked with salt in   serving
    their own fats or with specified oil. No pepper, con-
    diments or sauces. Gravies thickened with potato
    flour. (Garnish lamb chops and dried chicken with
    broiled pineapple, apricots or prunes.)(13)

Vegetables:

    (*a*) Any of those listed in this diet, cooked with salt, with-   ½ cup
    out pepper and served with prescribed oil or Sesame
    Spread.

    (*b*) White or sweet potato or yam baked, boiled, or fried in   1 med.
    prescribed oils. Sesame Spread and salt may be used.

    (*c*) Sweet potato or yam candied with brown sugar or   1 med.
    maple syrup and Sesame Spread.

Suggested Menu—(Continued)

LUNCH OR DINNER

Approximate amounts

Bread:
Choice of those suggested for breakfast.
Butter Substitute:
As suggested for breakfast.
Jams or Preserves:
Choice of those suggested for breakfast.
Desserts:
   (*a*) Fruit as suggested for breakfast.   ½ cup
   (*b*) Tapioca fruit pudding.(14)   ½ cup
   (*c*) Lemon, lime or pineapple flavored gelatin plain,   ½ cup
       whipped or with fruit added.
   (*d*) Pears baked with brown sugar.(15)   1 whole
   (*e*) Lemon, pineapple or apricot water ice made at   pear
       home.(16) (Commercial sherbets and ices contain
       milk, egg or other forbidden foods.)
   (Soy bean-lima bean-potato cookies, cakes or cup cakes
   as desired.)(17)
Beverage:
Choice of those suggested for breakfast.
Candies:
   (*a*) Candied grapefruit or lemon peel or glacéd pine-
       apple.(18) (Made at home.)
   (*b*) Dried prunes pitted and stuffed with lemon flavored
       fondant. (Made at home.)
   (*c*) Pure maple sugar candy.
   (*d*) Plain fondant may be made at home and flavored with
       the fruits on this diet.(19)
Between meals, if desired, the patient may have lime, lemon or pineapple
      gelatin, tapioca fruit pudding, canned fruits, cookies, cakes, cupcakes
      or candy made according to recipes in this volume.
This menu contains approximately 1227 calories.
Total for the day:

Calories	3225	Carbohydrate	368 grams	Ca	0.336 gram
		Protein	112 grams	P	1.398 grams
		Fat	145 grams	Fe	0.025 gram

Comments. The use of the elimination diets as summarized on page 155 and discussed in Chapter V must be accurately followed. Indicated vitamins and the addition of other foods after an adequate period of relief are there discussed. Specific directions for the addition of rice and corn are on page 201.

The exclusion of all cereal grains including wheat from this diet is due to the frequency of allergy to group allergens as well as to specific allergens in all cereal grains. (See page 62.) The tendency for legumes to produce "gas in the intestines" at times necessitates a change to the menu for Diets 1 and 2 on page 161. At time allergic symptoms arise to legumes.

Soy and lima bean flours must be pure and obtained from honest millers and merchants. Various recipes for bread, muffins, cookies, cake, pancakes and waffles indicated by numbers in the menus are found on page 238.

If Sesame oil is not obtainable, pure olive or soy bean oil (see page 96) may be used if no allergy is evident thereto. For content of Sesame Spread see page 156.

Diets 1 and 2 (Rowe)

Foods Allowed

Rice	Lemon
Corn	Grapefruit
Rye	Pears
Tapioca	Pineapple
Sweet potato or yam	Peaches
	Apricots
Rice Biscuit	Prunes
Rice bread	
Corn pone	Cane or beet sugar
Corn-rye muffins	Salt
Rye bread	Sesame oil
Ry-Krisp	Mazola oil
	Sesame Spread
Lettuce	Gelatin, plain
Chard	Lime, lemon or pineapple flavored gel-
Spinach	atin
Carrots	Maple syrup or syrup made with cane
Beets	sugar flavored with maple
Squash	Karo Corn Syrup
Asparagus	White vinegar
Artichoke	Vanilla extract
	Lemon extract
Lamb	Royal baking powder
Chicken (no hens)	Baking soda
Bacon	Cream of tartar

Suggested Menu

	BREAKFAST	Approximate amounts
Beverage:		
(*a*)	Grapefruit juice, fresh or canned.	1 cup
(*b*)	Pineapple, apricot, peach or prune juice, singly or mixed with grapefruit juice.	1 cup
Cereal or Cereal Substitute:		
(*a*)	Boiled brown or polished rice or cornmeal mush served with apricot, prune or peach juice or maple syrup.	½ cup
(*b*)	Corn or rice flakes, puffed rice or Rice Krispies served with grapefruit juice and sugar or with apricots, peaches, prunes or pears and the fruit juices.	1 cup
(*c*)	Cold boiled rice or sliced cold cornmeal mush fried in Mazola oil, sesame oil or bacon fat and served with maple or Karo syrup.	½ cup or 2 slices
(*d*)	Tapioca cooked with water or fruit juice and puréed apricots, peaches, prunes or pineapple. Serve hot.	½ cup

11

Suggested Menu—(Continued)

BREAKFAST

Meat:

		Approximate amounts
(a)	Bacon.	4 strips
(b)	Lamb chops, lamb patties with bacon, lamb or chicken croquettes.(3)	1 med. chop or equiv.
(c)	Lamb kidney or liver fried with bacon.	3 slices

Bread:

(a)	Corn pone.(20)	2 muffins
(b)	Corn-rice muffins.(21)	
(c)	Corn-rye muffins.(22)	
(d)	Rice biscuit.(23)	
(e)	Rice bread.(24)	2 thin slices
(f)	Ry-Krisp.(25)	
(g)	Corn and rice flour pancakes served with Karo or maple syrup and Sesame Spread.(26)	2 cakes

Butter Substitute:

Sesame Spread; salted, hydrogenated sesame oil or bacon grease.

Jams or Preserves:

(a)	Apricot, aprico-pineapple, peach or prune jam.(7)	2 tsp.
(b)	Lemon, grapefruit, or carrot marmalade.(8)	2 tsp.
(c)	Pear butter.(10b)	

Fruit:

(a)	Fresh or canned grapefruit, pears, pineapple, peaches, apricots or prunes	½ grapefruit 1 peach or pear
(b)	Cooked dried prunes. Lemon juice and sugar may be added as desired. Do not use dried peaches or apricots.	4 prunes

This menu contains approximately 956 calories.

LUNCH OR DINNER

Soup:

(a)	Lamb or chicken broth, clear or with rice, tapioca or prescribed vegetables added. Salt may be used in cooking but no other seasonings or condiments. (No canned soups or broths or any away from home.)	½ cup

Salad:

Any combination of vegetables or fruits listed in this diet, dressing made of Mazola or sesame oil, white vinegar or lemon juice, salt and sugar.

(Variations: [1] Lemon, lime or pineapple flavored gelatin with grated raw carrots and crushed pineapple. [2] Cooked sliced beets pickled in white vinegar seasoned with salt and sugar. [3] Cut tender young carrots into long thin strips and place in iced salted water for one-half hour. Use as a garnish for salads or as an appetizer.)

½ cup veg. or fruit
1 Tbsp. oil

Meat:

Approximate
amounts

   (a) Lamb—chops, roast, boiled tongue or stew with rice, corn or carrots as desired. Meat may be hot or cold. — 2 med. chops or equiv.

   (b) Chicken (no hens) may be fried, broiled, roasted or fricasseed. Use only rice flour, cornstarch or cornmeal to dredge chicken or thicken gravy. Fry in Sesame or Mazola oil, bacon or chicken fat. — ½ fryer or equiv.

   (c) Lamb or chicken (no hens) liver sautéed with bacon. — 3 slices

   (d) Lamb patties(3) or lamb or chicken croquettes.(27) (Garnish lamb chops and dried chicken with hot, broiled pineapple, apricots or prunes.)(13) — 2 med.

Vegetables:

   (a) Spinach, chard, carrots, beets, summer and winter squash, asparagus, artichokes or corn. Flavor with salt and bacon, sesame oil or Mazola oil or Sesame Spread. — ½ cup

   (b) Boiled brown or polished rice or cooked rice fried in bacon fat. — ½ cup

   (c) Baked, boiled or candied sweet potatoes and yams. — 1 med.

   (d) Hominy — ½ cup

Bread:

   (a) Corn Crisps with soup and salads.(28)

   (b) Choice of breads suggested for breakfast.

Butter Substitute:

As suggested for breakfast.

Jams or Preserves:

Choice of those suggested for breakfast.

Dessert:

   (a) Fruit as suggested for breakfast.

   (b) Rice fruit pudding with vanilla sauce.(29) — ½ cup

   (c) Tapioca fruit pudding.(14) — ½ cup

   (d) Lemon or lime flavored gelatin plain, whipped or with fruit added. — ½ cup

   (e) Pears baked with brown sugar.(15) — 1 pear

   (f) Rice cupcakes or corn and rice cookies.(30) — 1 cake

   (g) Lemon, pineapple or apricot water ice made at home. (16)

Beverage:

Grapefruit, peach, apricot, or pineapple juices or lemonade. — 1 cup

Candies:

   (a) Candied grapefruit or lemon peel, or glaced pineapple, made at home.(18) — 2 slices

   (b) Puffed rice candy or marshmallows made at home.(31) — 2 pieces

   (c) Dried prunes pitted and stuffed with lemon flavored fondant.(19)

   (d) Pure maple sugar candy.

This menu contains approximately 1193 calories.

Total for the day, 3342 calories.

Carbohydrate	325 gm.	Ca	0.319 gm.
Protein	110 gm.	P	1.511 gm.
Fat	178 gm.	Fe	0.022 gm.

NOTE.—The use of the elimination diets as summarized on page 155 and discussed in Chapter V must be accurately followed. These diets are legume-free and also exclude tomato and potato. The bakery products must be made according to numbered recipes (page 237) or by honest bakers according to such recipes. Calcium and vitamins must be given as suggested on page 147.

Elimination Diet 1 (Rowe)

Foods Allowed

Tapioca   Lamb
Rice

                 Sugar
Rice Biscuit   Salt
Rice bread   Sesame oil
                 Sesame Spread
Lettuce   Gelatin, plain
Chard   Lime and lemon flavored gelatin
Spinach   Maple syrup or syrup made with cane sugar
Carrots   flavored with maple
Sweet potato   Lemon extract
Yam   Vanilla extract
                 Royal baking powder
Lemon   Cream or tartar
Grapefruit   Baking soda
Pears

Suggested Menu

BREAKFAST

Beverage:
    (a) Grapefruit juice or lemonade with sugar added as desired. May be hot or cold. — ½ cup
    (b) Pear juice flavored with lemon — ½ cup

Cereal or Cereal Substitute:
    (a) Boiled brown or polished rice served hot with pear juice, maple syrup or syrup made with cane sugar flavored with maple. — ½ cup
    (b) Rice flakes, Rice Krispies or puffed rice served with pears and pear juice. — ¾ cup
    (c) Tapioca cooked in water and flavored with caramel or lemon juice and grated lemon rind and sugar.(2) — ½ cup

Meat:
    (a) Lamb chops or lamb patties.(3) — 1 med.
    (b) Lamb tongue served hot or cold. — 3 slices
    (c) Lamb liver fried in sesame oil — 2 slices

Bread:
    (a) Rice biscuits.(23) — 1 biscuit
    (b) Rice bread.(24) — 2 slices

Butter Substitute:
Sesame Spread or salted, hydrogenated sesame oil.

BREAKFAST

Jams or Preserves:
- (*a*) Lemon, grapefruit or carrot marmalade.(8)   2 tsp.
- (*b*) Pear butter.(10)   2 tsp.

Fruit:
- (*a*) Sectioned or half grapefruit, fresh or canned.   ¾ cup
- (*b*) Fresh or canned pears.   2 halves

This meal contains approximately 747 calories.

LUNCH OR DINNER

Soup:
Lamb broth, clear or with tapioca, rice and carrots added.   1 cup
 No pepper, spices, flavors, and no canned soup.

Salad:
- (*a*) Hearts of lettuce with sesame oil and lemon juice   ¼ head
 dressing   1 Tbsp. oil
- (*b*) Vegetable salad of lettuce, chopped tender spinach   ½ cup veg.
 leaves and diced cooked carrots. Serve with sesame   1 Tbsp. oil
 oil and lemon juice.
- (*c*) Sectioned grapefruit or halves of pears served on   ½ pear
 shredded lettuce.
- (*d*) Grated raw carrot, sectioned grapefruit, or halves of   ½ cup
 pears molded in lime or lemon flavored gelatin.(32)

Meat:
- (*a*) Lamb roast and chops.   2 med.
     chops
- (*b*) Stew made of lamb, rice and carrots. Thicken gravy   1 cup
 with rice flour.
- (*c*) Lamb kidney, liver and boiled tongue.   3 slices

Vegetables:
- (*a*) Boiled brown or polished rice. Cold cooked rice may   ½ cup
 be fried in sesame oil.
- (*b*) Baked, boiled or candied sweet potatoes or yams. Use   1 med.
 sesame oil and brown sugar or maple syrup to candy
 the sweet potatoes.
- (*c*) Steamed spinach, chard or carrots. Flavor with salt   3 Tbsp.
 and sesame oil.

Bread:
Rice bread or rice biscuit.(24)   2 slices

Butter Substitute:
As suggested for breakfast.   1 Tbsp.

Jams or Preserves:
Choice of those suggested for breakfast.   2 tsp.

Desserts:
- (*a*) Pears baked with maple syrup or brown sugar.(15)   1 whole
     pear
- (*b*) Rice cupcakes or rice cookies.(30)   1 cake
- (*c*) Lemon or lime flavored gelatin; plain, whipped or with   ½ cup
 added grapefruit or pears.

Suggested Menu—(Continued)

LUNCH OR DINNER

	Approximate Amounts

Desserts:

(d) Tapioca flavored with caramel or lemon juice and lemon rind and sugar.(2)   ½ cup

(e) Rice pudding flavored with lemon juice and rind, served with lemon sauce.(33)   ½ cup

(f) Lemon water ice made at home.(16) (Commercial ices or sherbets contain milk or eggs.)

Beverage:

(a) Grapefruit juice or lemonade.   1 cup

(b) Pear juice.   1 cup

Candies:

(a) Candied lemon or grapefruit peel.(18)   3 slices

(b) Puffed rice candy or marshmallows made at home.(31)   2 pieces

(c) Maple sugar candy, pure.

(d) Fondant.(19)

This menu contains approximately 1328 calories. Total for the day, 3403 calories.

Carbohydrate	336 gm.	Ca	0.350 gm.
Protein	132 gm.	P	1.359 gm.
Fat	170 gm.	Fe	0.207 gm.

NOTE.—The use of the elimination diets as summarized on page 155 and discussed in Chapter V must be accurately followed. Numbers in menu refer to recipes (see page 237).

Elimination Diet 2 (Rowe)

Foods Allowed

Corn	Chicken
Rye	Bacon
Corn pone	Sugar
Corn rye muffin	Salt
Rye bread	Mazola oil
Ry-Krisp	Sesame oil
	Sesame Spread
Beets	Gelatin, plain or flavored with pineapple
Squash	
Asparagus	Karo Corn Syrup
Artichoke	Maple syrup or syrup made with cane sugar flavored with maple
Pineapple	White vinegar
Peach	Vanilla extract
Apricot	Royal baking powder
Prune	Cream of tartar
	Baking soda

Suggested Menu

BREAKFAST

		Approximate
Beverage:		*amounts*

Beverage:
- (a) Pineapple or prune juice. — ½ cup
- (b) Apricot, peach and pineapple juices mixed. — ½ cup

Cereal:
- (a) Cornflakes served with apricots, peaches or prunes and juice. — 1 cup / 4 prunes
- (b) Cornmeal mush served hot with maple or Karo syrup. — ½ cup
- (c) Sliced cold cornmeal mush fried in Mazola oil or bacon fat served with syrup and strips of bacon. — 3 slices / 4 strips

Meat:
- (a) Bacon. — 4 strips
- (b) Chicken croquettes.(27) — 2
- (c) Sautéed chicken livers with bacon. — 3 Tbsp.

Bread:
- (a) Corn pone.(20) — 2 slices
- (b) Corn and rye muffins.(22) — 2 muffins
- (c) Rye bread.(34) — 2 thin slices
- (d) Ry-Krisp.(25) — 2 wafers

Butter Substitute:
Sesame Spread; salted, hydrogenated sesame oil or bacon grease. — 1 Tbsp.

Jams or Preserves:
Peach, prune, apricot or pineapple-apricot jam. — 2 tsp.

Fruit:
- (a) Fresh or canned pineapple, peaches, apricots or prunes. — 2 slices
- (b) Stewed dried prunes. Do not use dried apricots or peaches. — 4 prunes

This menu contains approximately 895 calories.

LUNCH OR DINNER

Soup:
Chicken broth. (No pepper, seasonings and no canned or restaurant broth.) — ½ cup

Salad:
- (a) Any combination of artichoke hearts, beets or asparagus with Mazola or sesame oil and white vinegar. — 1 cup mixed veg or equiv.
- (b) Cold sliced beets marinated in white vinegar, seasoned with salt and sugar. — 5 slices
- (c) Any combination of pineapple, peaches, apricots or prunes. Any of these fruits may be molded in plain or pineapple flavored gelatin. — ½ cup

Meat:
- (a) Chicken—roasted, fried, broiled or fricasseed. Use cornmeal or rye flour for dredging and cornstarch for thickening gravy. Mazola oil, sesame oil, bacon or chicken fat can be used for frying. — ½ fryer or equiv.
- (b) Chicken croquettes.(27) — 2 med.
- (c) Sautéed chicken livers. — ½ cup

Suggested Menu—(Continued)

LUNCH OR DINNER

	Approximate amounts
Vegetables:	
(*a*) Fresh or canned beets, corn, summer and winter squash, asparagus and artichokes.	½ cup
(*b*) Hominy	½ cup
Bread:	
(*a*) Choice of those suggested for breakfast.	
(*b*) Corn Crisps—serve with salad or soup.(28)	2
Butter Substitute:	
As suggested for breakfast.	1 Tbsp.
Jams or Preserves:	
Choice of those suggested for breakfast.	2 tsp.
Desserts:	
(*a*) Fruits as suggested for breakfast.	
(*b*) Rye coffee cake.(35)	2 cookies
(*c*) Cornstarch pudding with crushed fruit.(36)	½ cup
(*d*) Jellied prunes and pineapple.(37)	4 prunes
(*e*) Plain or pineapple flavored gelatin with fruits listed in this diet.	½ cup
Beverage:	
Choice of those suggested for breakfast.	
Candies:	
(*a*) Candied pineapple.(18)	1 slice
(*b*) Dried pitted prunes stuffed with candied pineapple or vanilla flavored fondant.(19)	2 prunes

This menu contains approximately 1036 calories.

Total for the day: Calories 2968.

Carbohydrate	322 gm.	Ca	0.290 gm.
Protein	89 gm.	P	1.401 gm.
Fat	147 gm.	Fe	0.019 gm.

NOTE.—The use of the elimination diets as summarized on page 155 and discussed in Chapter V must be accurately followed. Addition of extra vitamins is there discussed. Numbers in menus refer to recipes (see page 237).

Elimination Diet 3 (Rowe)

Foods Allowed

Tapioca	Beef
White potato	Bacon
Lima bean-potato bread	Sugar
Soy bean-lima bean bread	Salt
Soy bean-potato-tapioca bread	Sesame oil
	Soy bean oil
Tomato	Sesame Spread

Carrots

Lima beans

Soy beans

String beans

Peas

Lemons

Grapefruit

Peaches

Apricots

Gelatin, plain

Lime or lemon flavored gelatin

Maple syrup or syrup made with cane
   sugar flavored with maple

Vanilla extract

Lemon extract

Royal baking powder

Baking soda

Cream of tartar

Suggested Menu

	BREAKFAST	*Approximate amounts*
Beverage:		
	(a) Grapefruit juice or lemonade with sugar as desired.	½ cup
	(b) Tomato juice.	½ cup
Cereal Substitute:		
	(a) Tapioca cooked with apricot or peach juice and puréed fruit.(1)	½ cup
	(b) Tapioca cooked in water, sweetened with sugar and flavored with lemon juice and grated lemon rind, caramel, brown sugar or maple syrup.(2)	½ cup
Meat:		
	(a) Bacon	4 slices
	(b) Beefsteak or beef patties.	2 med. pats
	(c) Calves or beef liver and bacon.	2 slices
	(d) Boiled beef tongue, cooked plain.	2 slices
	(Hashed brown potatoes cooked in prescribed oils can be served with meats.)	½ cup
Bread:		
	(a) Lima bean-soy bean bread or muffins.	2 thin slices
	(b) Soy bean-potato bread or muffins	2 thin slices
	(c) Soy bean pancakes served with maple syrup or syrup made of cane sugar flavored with maple.(6)	4 medium
Butter Substitute:		
	Sesame Spread; salted, hydrogenated sesame oil or bacon grease.	1 Tbsp.
Jams or Preserves:		
	(a) Lemon, grapefruit or carrot marmalade.(8)	2 tsp.
	(b) Peach or apricot jam.	2 tsp.
	(c) Tomato preserves flavored with lemon.(9)	2 tsp.
Fruit:		
	(a) Fresh or canned grapefruit.	½ grapefruit
	(b) Peaches or apricots (fresh or canned).	1 peach or 3 apricots
	(c) Sliced tomatoes with sugar.	

This menu contains approximately 656 calories.

Suggested Menu—(Continued)

LUNCH OR DINNER

Approximate amounts

Soup:

   (*a*) Beef broth clear (not canned) or with tapioca, carrots,   ½ cup
tomatoes, lima beans or peas (no pepper).

   (*b*) Lima bean soup flavored with bacon.(11)   ½ cup

   (*c*) Vegetable broth made with tomatoes, carrots, lima   ½ cup
beans, string beans and diced potatoes.(38)

Salad:

   (*a*) Vegetable salad of any combination of tomatoes, car-   ½ cup
rots, lima beans, string beans and peas. Serve with
French dressing of sesame oil, lemon juice and salt.

   (*b*) Fruit salad of grapefruit, peaches and apricots. (Use   ¾ cup
lemon or lime flavored gelatin with any of the above
listed fruits or vegetables. Cut tender young carrots
into long thin strips and place in iced salted water for
one-half hour. Use as a garnish for salads or as an
appetizer.)

Meat:

   (*a*) Beef served as steak, roast, patties or meat loaf.(39)   Liberal

   (*b*) Beef stew with white potatoes, carrots, tomatoes, peas,   serving
lima beans or string beans. Thicken gravy with   of meat
potato flour.

   (*c*) Calves or beef liver and bacon.   3 slices

   (*d*) Boiled calves or beef tongue, cooked plain.   3 slices.

Vegetables:

   (*a*) White potatoes may be baked, boiled, riced, hash   1 med.
browned or French fried. Use only sesame or soy bean
oil.

   (*b*) Fresh or canned tomatoes, carrots, lima beans, string   ½ cup
beans, peas and soy beans.

Bread:

  Choice of those suggested for breakfast.

Butter Substitute:

  As suggested for breakfast.   1 Tbsp.

Jams or Preserves:

  Choice of those suggested for breakfast.   2 tsp.

Dessert:

   (*a*) Fruit as suggested for breakfast.

   (*b*) Tapioca pudding made with apricots or peaches.(14)   ½ cup

   (*c*) Lemon or apricot water ice made at home.(16)   ½ cup

   (*d*) Lima bean or soy bean cookies or cup cakes.(17)   2 cookies

Beverage:

   (*a*) Grapefruit juice or lemonade with sugar as desired.   ½ cup

   (*b*) Tomato juice.   ½ cup

Candies:

   (*a*) Candied grapefruit or lemon peel.(18)   2 slices

   (*b*) Fondant flavored with vanilla, lemon or apricot.(19)   2 pieces

   (*c*) Pure maple sugar candy.

This menu contains approximately 1267 calories.

Total for the day: Calories 3190.

Carbohydrate	330 gm.	Ca	0.300 gm.
Protein	105 gm.	P	1.203 gm.
Fat	161 gm.	Fe	0.024 gm.

NOTE.—The use of the elimination diets as summarized on page 155 and discussed in Chapter V must be accurately followed. Indicated vitamins are there discussed. Numbers in menus refer to recipes on page 237.

FRUIT–FREE ELIMINATION DIETS

Certain food sensitive patients are allergic to several fruits and at times apparently to all fruits. Some individuals can take cooked but not uncooked ones. Some are sensitive to the skins and not to the meat of the fruits. At times allergy to fruits is extremely specific, being restricted to one species of melon, apple, or grape.

Fruit sensitive patients most frequently develop urticaria and less often angioneurotic edema and gastro-intestinal manifestations. Generalized joint swellings and at times soreness and stiffness may arise. A further discussion of these manifestations from fruit allergy is in Chapter IV.

Certain patients with such fruit allergy develop definite symptoms, especially in the gastro-intestinal tract when cevitamic acid is taken. This apparent allergy to the synthetic vitamin C in fruit sensitive patients is being discussed in a forthcoming article by the writer. It necessitates the eating of various vegetables rich in vitamin C as shown in published tables. (See page 203.)

Fruit–free, Cereal–free Elimination Diets 1, 2 and 3 (Rowe)

Foods Allowed

Tapioca
White potato
Sweet potato or yam

Lima bean-potato bread
Soy bean-lima bean bread
Soy bean-potato-tapioca bread

Chard
Spinach*
Carrots
Beets
Squash
Asparagus
Artichoke
Tomato*
Lima beans
String beans
Peas

Lamb
Beef
Chicken (no hens)
Bacon

Cane or beet sugar
Sesame oil
Soy bean oil
Sesame Spread
Gelatin
Salt
Maple syrup or syrup made with cane
   sugar flavored with maple
Vanilla extract
Royal baking powder
Baking soda
Cream of tartar
White vinegar

* Should be eliminated if allergy thereto is suggested by history. (See Comments.)

Suggested Menu

BREAKFAST

	Approximate amounts
Beverage:	
Tomato or carrot juice (canned and unspiced).	5 to 8 oz.
Cereal Substitute:	
(a) Tapioca (Instant or Pearl) cooked with water and maple syrup, brown or caramelized sugar.(2)	1 large helping
(b) Pancakes or waffles made of soy and lima bean flours, served with Sesame Spread and maple syrup.(6)	4 med. cakes
Meat:	
(a) Bacon	4 slices
(b) Lamb or beef—chops, steak, patties, or tongue (unspiced).	2 med. chops or equiv.
(c) Lamb, calves or beef liver and bacon.	
Bread:	
(a) Bread made of any combination of soy bean, lima bean, and potato flours and tapioca.(4)	2 to 4 slices toasted
(b) Muffins made of above flours.(5)	2 muffins
Butter Substitute:	
Sesame Spread, bacon grease, or salted, hydrogenated sesame oil.	1 Tbsp.
Jams or Preserves:	
Tomato or carrot preserves (made without lemon juice), or maple syrup.	2 tsp.
Fruit Substitute:	
Tomato, fresh cooked or canned, served with sugar if desired.	½ cup

This menu contains approximately 587 calories.

LUNCH OR DINNER

	Approximate amounts
Soup:	
(a) Broth made of lamb, beef, or chicken (no hens), served clear with tapioca or cooked with vegetables listed above. (No pepper or spices, no canned soups.)	1 cup
(b) Lima bean or split pea purée, flavored with bacon.(11)	1 cup
Salad:	
(a) Any combination of the cooked vegetables listed in this diet. Dressing may be made of soy bean or sesame oil, white vinegar, salt, and a little sugar.	1 cup mixed veg. 1 Tbsp. oil
(b) Molded salad using plain gelatin and vegetables previously listed. French dressing as in (a).	
Meat:	
(a) Lamb and beef—chops, steak, ground plain meat, roast (hot or cold) cooked with salt in their own fats or with specified oil. No pepper, condiments or sauces. Gravies thickened with potato flour.	Av. liberal serving
(b) Beef, lamb or calves tongue and liver cooked as above.	
(c) Chicken (no hens) may be roasted, fried, broiled or fricasseed. Sesame or soy bean oil or Sesame Spread and salt may be used. Thicken gravy with potato flour.	½ broiler or fryer or equiv.

Vegetables:
- (*a*) Any of those listed in this diet, cooked with salt, without pepper, and served with sesame or soy bean oil or Sesame Spread.   4 Tbsp. veg.
- (*b*) White or sweet potato or yam, baked, boiled, or fried in above oils. Sesame Spread and salt may be used.   1 med. sized potato
- (*c*) Sweet potato or yam candied with brown sugar or maple syrup and Sesame Spread.

Bread:
Choice of those suggested for breakfast.

Butter Substitute:
As suggested for breakfast.

Jams or Preserves:
As at breakfast.

Dessert:
- (*a*) Tapioca cooked as at breakfast.   Av. serving
- (*b*) Cookies, cake or cupcakes made of any combination of soy, lima, and potato flours and tapioca.(17)   2 cookies or 1 cupcake

Beverage:
Tomato or carrot juice (canned and unspiced).   5 to 8 oz.

This menu contains approximately 1263 calories.

Total for the day: Calories 3112.

Carbohydrate	264 gm.	Ca	0.370 gm.
Protein	136 gm.	P	1.459 gm.
Fat	168 gm.	Fe	0.024 gm.

Comments: The directions for the use of the elimination diets as summarized on page 155 and discussed in Chapter V must be accurately followed. When weight maintenance is important, special attention to the proper intake of calorie-carrying foods included in this diet and as discussed on pages 146 and 207 is most necessary.

When the allergic manifestation has been absent for an adequate period, then various foods, one every five to seven days, can be added. The addition of fruits should be delayed for one to three months. It may be found that all fruits reproduce symptoms or that cooked fruits are tolerated. At times tolerance to such allergenic fruits returns only after their elimination for weeks or months and at times fruit allergy persists for years. Possible hyposensitization to fruits in such cases is discussed on page 59. At times fruit-sensitive patients are also allergic to tomato. This necessitates its exclusion. Spinach allergy may occur. The use of additional calcium and vitamins and especially of vitamin C is discussed in directions for the use of diets on pages 147 and 155. Possible allergy to cevitamic acid may exist.

Fruit-free Elimination Diets 1 and 2 (Rowe)

Foods Allowed

Rice	Lamb
Corn	Chicken
Rye	Bacon
Tapioca	
Sweet potato or yam	Sugar
	Salt

Fruit-free Elimination Diets 1 and 2 (Rowe)—*(Continued)*

Foods Allowed

Rice bread	Sesame oil
Corn pone	Mazola oil
Corn-rye muffins	Sesame Spread
Rye bread	Gelatin
Ry-Krisp	White vinegar
	Maple syrup or syrup made with
Chard	cane sugar flavored with maple
Spinach*	Karo syrup
Carrots	Vanilla extract
Beets	Royal baking powder
Squash	Baking soda
Asparagus	Cream of tartar
Artichoke	
Tomato*	

Suggested Menu

BREAKFAST

Approximate amounts

Beverage:
  (a) Tomato juice (canned and unspiced).   5 to 8 oz.
  (b) Carrot juice (canned).
Cereal:
  (a) Boiled brown or polished rice or cooked cornmeal   ½ cup
      served with sugar, granulated or brown, maple syrup
      or Karo corn syrup
  (b) Rice Krispies or corn flakes served as above.   ¾ cup dry
                                                          flakes
  (c) Cold cooked rice or corn meal fried in Mazola oil,
      sesame oil or bacon fat, served with maple syrup or
      Karo corn syrup.
Meat:
  (a) Bacon   4 slices
  (b) Lamb—chops, croquettes, patties or tongue.(27)   1 med. chop
  (c) Lamb liver and bacon.   or equiv.
Bread:
  (a) Corn pone.(20)   2 muffins
  (b) Corn-rice muffins.(21)
  (c) Corn-rye muffins.(22)
  (d) Rice bread.(24)   2 to 4 slices
  (e) Rye bread.(34)   toasted
  (f) Ry-Krisp.(25)
Butter Substitute:
  Sesame Spread, bacon grease; or salted, hydrogenated   1 Tbsp.
      sesame oil.
Jams or Preserves:
  Tomato or carrot preserves (made without lemon juice).   2 tsp.
Fruit Substitute:
  Tomato, fresh cooked or canned, served with sugar if   ½ cup
      desired.

This menu contains approximately 526 calories.

* Should be eliminated if allergy thereto is suggested by history. (See Comments on page 173.)

LUNCH OR DINNER

Approximate amounts

Salad:

(a) Combination salad containing any of the vegetables listed above. White vinegar, sesame or Mazola oil, and salt may be used as a dressing.

1 cup mixed veg.
1 Tbsp. oil

(b) Molded salad using plain gelatin and vegetables listed above. French dressing as above.

Soup:

(a) Broth made of lamb or chicken (no hens), cooked with vegetables included in this diet and thickened with rice flour, cornstarch or tapioca. May be seasoned with salt but no pepper or condiments may be used.

1 cup

(b) Plain chicken broth with rice, seasoned with salt. (No canned or restaurant soups.)

Meat:

(a) Lamb chops, roast, tongue, liver, or lamb stew with rice, corn, carrots, beets and tomato, cooked in their own fats or with sesame or Mazola oil or Sesame Spread

2 med. chops or equiv.

(b) Chicken (no hens) may be roasted, fried, broiled, stewed. Sesame or Mazola oil or Sesame Spread and salt may be used. Dredge chicken in rice flour. Thicken gravy with rice flour or cornstarch.

$\frac{1}{2}$ broiler or fryer or equiv.

Vegetables:

(a) Sweet potato or yam, boiled, baked, candied, or fried in specified oils or Sesame Spread.

1 med. sized potato

(b) Any vegetables listed in this diet, cooked with salt, without pepper, and served with Sesame Spread or sesame or Mazola oil.

4 Tbsp.

(c) Hominy or steamed rice.

Bread:

Choice of those suggested for breakfast.

Butter Substitute:

As at breakfast.

Jams or Preserves:

As at breakfast.

Dessert:

(a) Cold cooked rice or cornmeal fried in prescribed oils served with butter substitute and maple or corn syrup, or vanilla pudding sauce.

Av. helping

(b) Tapioca cooked with water and granulated, brown, or caramelized sugar, or maple or corn syrup.(2)

(c) Rice or rye cookies.(30–35)

Beverages:

(a) Tomato juice.

5 to 8 oz.

(b) Carrot juice.

This menu contains approximately 1021 calories.

Total for the day: Calories 2568.

Carbohydrate	230 gm.	Ca	0.256 gm.
Protein	133 gm.	P	1.696 gm.
Fat	124 gm.	Fe	0.025 gm.

Comments: The same suggestions apply to this diet as are detailed on page 173.

MEALS EATEN AWAY FROM HOME IN HOTELS, RESTAURANTS, TRAINS, OR FRIENDS' HOMES

Adherence to an elimination diet is usually possible away from home if the patient insists on accuracy of selection and cooking of foods. The menus which are detailed below include plain foods such as dry cereals or plain cooked cornmeal or rice, fruit juices, plain unseasoned and unbuttered vegetables, baked or boiled potatoes in their jackets, plain cooked meats without gravies, pepper, flavors, or sauces, plain fresh or canned fruits, Ry-Krisp or bread or cookies carried by the patient from his home or from his honest baker. In restaurant, hotel, or dining car, such foods can be ordered. Special insistence is always necessary to obtain unseasoned meats, cooked without butter or gravy, and plain vegetables. If such are not served, the patient should request others. At no time should he eat food which he suspects contains a forbidden ingredient such as milk or its products, wheat, egg, or other excluded food. He can always eat more of the correctly selected foods or eat in one to four hours thereafter of foods allowed in his diet. If he continues to eat at one hotel or restaurant, careful explanation to waitress, waiter, and if possible, to the cook will insure greater accuracy. However, the patient's vigilance is always necessary to protect against carelessness or occasional mistakes. If he can eat where he can see the food actually cooked, errors are less likely.

Eating at friends' homes is always difficult. Unless the friend thoroughly understands the patient's diet and the reasons behind it, mistakes are inevitable. Therefore, it is best to eat before going to such homes or to limit the food to simple articles such as sliced tomato, plain meat and vegetables, baked or boiled potato, and canned or fresh fruit. While diet trial is continuing, no slight mistake should be allowed, even though it is embarassing to the patient and host.

Patients who eat in boarding houses must explain their menus to the cook and attendants. For a small additional sum, extra attention is usually available so that accurate meals are provided. If such are not possible, then the patient should find another boarding house before embarking on a period of diet trial. Slight inaccuracies make such diet trial worthless.

When meals must be eaten away from home as described above, the patient should have extra bakery products obtained from bakers approved and supervised by his physician, fresh or canned fruit, and possibly cold meat in his room if adequate regular meals are not obtainable. Undesirable weight loss should not be permitted, and can be prevented, as discussed on page 155 by eating extra prescribed food as outlined on page 207. Nutrition must be protected as discussed on page 146 at all times.

Cereal–free Elimination Diets 1, 2 and 3 (Rowe)

(EATEN AWAY FROM HOME)

Foods Allowed

Tapioca	Lemon
White potato	Grapefruit
Sweet potato or yam	Pears
	Pineapple
Lima bean-potato bread	Peach
Soy bean-lima bean bread	Apricot
Soy bean-potato-tapioca bread .	Prune
Lettuce	Cane or beet sugar
Chard	Soy bean oil
Spinach	Sesame oil
Carrots	Sesame Spread
Beets	Salt
Squash	Gelatin, plain, or flavored with
Asparagus	lime, lemon or pineapple
Artichokes	Maple syrup or syrup made with
Tomato	sugar flavored with maple
Lima beans	White vinegar
String beans	Vanilla extract
Peas	Lemon extract
	Royal baking powder
Lamb	Baking soda
Beef	Cream of tartar
Chicken (no hens)	
Bacon	

Suggested Menu

BREAKFAST

Beverage:
  Grapefruit juice—5 to 7 ounces, with sugar. Other fruit juices listed
   below may be used.
Cereal Substitute:
  (a) Tapioca, cooked with pear, peach, apricot and sugar. (See Comments.)
  (b) Potatoes—white or sweet—baked or boiled, or fried in sesame or
   pure soy bean oil.
Bread:
  Soy-lima or potato-lima bread, muffins, or other bakery products. (See
   Comments.) (Jam or jelly of fruits on diet or maple syrup may be
   used on the bread.)
12

Suggested Menu—(Continued)

BREAKFAST

Meat:

Bacon—several slices (fried in clean pan alone.)

Fruit:

Pears, peaches, apricots, prunes, or pineapple—canned, cooked dried, or fresh.

Water.

LUNCH OR DINNER

Salad:

Made of vegetables or fruits listed below. Dressing of sesame or soy bean oil with lemon or white vinegar and salt may be used. (See note below.)

Meat:

Lamb, mutton or beef—steak, chops, roast (hot or cold), cooked in their own fat or with prescribed oils and salt. (No gravy.)

Vegetables:

Lettuce, tomato, spinach, chard, carrots, squash, asparagus, peas, artichokes, beets, string beans, and lima beans. (Prescribed oils, lemon, white vinegar, and salt may be used.)

Potatoes:

White or sweet potatoes or yams, baked or boiled, or fried in sesame or pure soy bean oil.

Bread:

As at breakfast.

Dessert:

Fruits or tapioca as at breakfast.

Beverages:

Grapefruit, pear, peach, apricot, pineapple, or tomato juices.

Water.

Comments: 1. The use of this elimination diet as summarized on page 155 and discussed in Chapter V must be accurately followed.

2. Since cereals are excluded, tapioca cooked with prescribed fruits and sugar and water is the only cereal substitute. This can be made rapidly from instant tapioca by any cook. Clean utensils free of all traces of other foods are essential.

3. If tapioca is not available, then potato may be eaten as a breakfast starch. If weight maintenance is not essential, these starches may be omitted.

4. Bread and bakery products must be made of soy, lima, or potato flour, according to recipes in this volume, at home or by honest bakers supervised by the physician. (See page 237.) They should be carried to the meal by the patient.

5. Sesame oil, obtained from the Globe Milling Company, California, or other dependable sources, may be brought and left for future use at hotel or restaurant or carried by the patient. If soy bean oil is used, it must be pure.

6. No hotel, restaurant, or canned soups are allowed.

7. Meats, vegetables, and potatoes must be cooked plain, salt being added by the patient.

8. Fruit salad in cans is permissible. If such contains a few grapes, it can be taken.

9. Extra vitamins and calcium should be prescribed by the physician to assure nutritional protection. Proper weight maintenance, if necessary, by extra amounts of the calorie-carrying foods is important. (See page 207.)

10. The physician must be assured of adequate nutrition in the patient and must supervise the accuracy of this diet trial. (See page 148.)

Elimination Diets 1 and 2—with Cereals (Rowe)

(Eaten Away From Home)

Foods Allowed

Rice	Lemon
Corn	Grapefruit
Rye	Pears
Tapioca	Pineapple
Sweet potato or yam	Peaches
	Apricots
Rice Biscuit	Prunes
Rice bread	
Corn pone	Cane or beet sugar
Corn-rye muffins	Salt
Rye bread	Sesame oil
Ry-Krisp	Mazola oil
	Sesame Spread
Lettuce	Gelatin, plain
Chard	Lime, lemon or pineapple flavored
Spinach	gelatin
Carrots	Maple syrup or syrup made with
Beets	cane sugar flavored with maple
Squash	Karo Corn Syrup
Asparagus	White vinegar
Artichoke	Vanilla extract
	Lemon extract
Lamb	Royal baking powder
Chicken (no hens)	Baking soda
Bacon	Cream of tartar

Suggested Menu

Breakfast

Beverage:
Grapefruit juice—5 to 6 ounces, with sugar.
Cereal:
  (a) Cornflakes
  (b) Rice flakes or Rice Krispies.
  (c) Cooked cornmeal.
  (d) Boiled rice.
  (All served with the juices of grapefruit, pear, peach, apricot or prunes
     with sugar or with maple syrup.)

Elimination Diets 1 and 2—with Cereals (Rowe)—*(Continued)*

(Eaten Away From Home)

Foods Allowed

Bread:
(*a*) Ry-Krisp.
(*b*) Rice, corn, or rye breads, muffins, or other bakery products brought from home or from supervised bakers made from recipes in this volume.

Jellies or Jams:
Those of fruits on the diet may be used. (No butter allowed.)

Meat:
Bacon—several slices.

Fruit:
Pear, peach, pineapple, prunes—canned, cooked dried or fresh (peeled).

Lunch or Dinner

Salad:
Made of plain vegetables (listed below). Dressing of Mazola, pure olive or sesame oil with lemon or white vinegar and salt. (No cottonseed oil should be used.)

Meat:
(*a*) Beef or lamb—chops, steak, or roasts (hot or cold) cooked in their own fats with salt. No pepper or spices. No gravies.
(*b*) Tongue or liver may be used, cooked plain as above.

Vegetables:
Lettuce, tomato, spinach, chard, carrots, squash, asparagus, peas, artichokes, beets, string beans, and lima beans. (Prescribed oil, lemon and salt only may be used.)

Potatoes:
White or sweet, or yams, boiled, baked, or fried only in proper oil. (Sesame Spread, but no milk, butter, or flour can be used.)

Bread:
Bread, cookies, and other bakery products as at breakfast.

Fruit:
As at breakfast.

Beverages:
Pineapple, grapefruit, apricot, peach, pear, or tomato juice.

Comments: 1. The use of this elimination diet as summarized on page 155 and discussed in Chapter V, must be accurately followed.

2. Grapefruit juice, preferably fresh, can be obtained in most areas. This amount assures proper vitamin C for the day. Other prescribed fruit or tomato juices may be taken. If grapefruit juice is not available, additional vitamin C may be required.

3. Ry-Krisp (Ralston) contains only 100 per cent rye flour and salt. Any other bread or bakery product must be brought by the patient to the meal and must be made at home or by honest, supervised bakers as discussed on page 149 from recipes in this book.

4. No restaurant, hotel, or canned soups can be taken since they contain pepper, varying spices, and other forbidden foods.

5. Meats, vegetables, and potatoes must be cooked plain without butter, milk, or pepper. Salt may be added by the patient. Sesame or soy bean oil should be brought to meal by patient. The ingredients in ordinary salad oils are difficult to determine.

6. The patient must not eat or taste any food suspected of containing any food, flavor, coloring or spice not allowed on his diet.

7. Clean spoons and cooking utensils advised on page 155 are imperative.

8. The physician must supervise the accuracy of this diet trial as discussed on page 148.

Fruit–free Elimination Diets 1, 2 and 3, and Fruit–free, Cereal–free Elimination Diets 1, 2 and 3

(Eaten Away From Home)

Menus for such diets are similar to those outlined on pages 171 to 175. The physician, dietitian, or patient, should write out the diet to be followed. The advice and precautions given in the former menus and also in the diets for hotels, restaurants, etc., given on pages 150, 173, 176, are most important to follow.

Since fruits are out of these diets, more of the tapioca cooked with sugar (see page 237), more of the vegetables and potatoes and allowed bakery products will be necessary as stressed in the fruit-free menus on pages 171 to 175. Proper nutrition, vitamins, and weight must be maintained.

OTHER SUPPLEMENTAL ELIMINATION DIETS

The use of supplemental elimination diets may be advisable as discussed on page 151, in those patients suspected of food allergy who do not respond to the routine elimination diets already detailed in this chapter.

1. Occasional patients are allergic to one or all mammalian meats. If fowl or fish are not suspected, they can be included in the trial diet. Milk, also, may be used unless evidence of possible allergy is quite definite. Possible tolerance for goat's milk and not for cow's milk was noted on page 200. If all animal proteins are under suspicion, then for a two or three week period of diet trial, the protein metabolism can be protected by increased amounts of the legumes (especially soy beans) as used in the cereal-free diets (see pages 158 to 160.)

If a diet of this type is prescribed, the physician, dietitian, or patient must prepare a detailed menu which contains enough food to assure regular meals which meet nutritional requirements. Additional vitamins and calcium are required.

2. A rare patient is apparently sensitive to all fruits and vegetables or can only tolerate two or three vegetables or, possibly, one or two fruits. At times, allergy to other common allergenic

foods, such as milk, egg, cereal grains, and fish is also present. Then, a diet containing tapioca, potatoes, beef, or lamb, and 2 or 3 vegetables, may be necessary for diet trial. If milk is not suspected, its use is most valuable in such possible vegetable and fruit sensitive individuals. With proper diet trial of this type, more definite suggestions about possible allergy to various foods can be obtained and a few foods may be found to produce little or no allergic reactivity. As such a diet is followed, increased tolerance for other vegetables and, possibly, for cooked fruits and other foods, becomes apparent. In these patients, hyposensitization with antigens containing important vegetable and fruit allergens occasionally may be helpful, as discussed on page 59.

In any of these diets, the physician's constant supervision is most necessary. The patient must have a list of the foods to be eaten. Carefully arranged, explicit menus must be provided. Usually, the same foods must be ingested at each meal. The justification for the monotony rests in the possible relief of the patient's symptoms, often invaliding and chronic in nature. The fact that Orientals usually live on limited diets such as rice, a few vegetables, fish, and pork, may offer some solace to the rare allergic patient whose problem justifies such limited elimination diets. The time such a diet must be followed is discussed on page 141.

The physician must prescribe proper vitamins which will satisfy the patient's requirements. Extra calcium must be given, if necessary. Proper weight must be protected with adequate calories, as stressed on page 207.

ELIMINATION DIETS FOR INFANTS AND YOUNG CHILDREN

Certain children are relieved of their allergic manifestations by the exclusion of foods to which aversions or obvious disagreements are present, or to which definite scratch reactions occur. Too often, false positive or negative reactions are obtained as discussed on page 13, and elimination diets are required for the adequate study of possible food sensitizations.

Until symptoms are relieved, it is best in nearly every case to exclude foods which commonly produce allergy, namely milk, egg, wheat, orange, banana, apple, fish, nuts, and several others. At first, because of group or specific allergens in cereal grains other than wheat, they are also excluded.

To meet protein requirements, soy bean preparations are available, especially in infancy.   The soy-milk formula, as printed on page 187, contains protein, calcium, phosphorus, and calories as contained in an equal amount of milk. Sobee is a powder containing such ingredients and can be added to water to make a milk substitute. Mull-Soy, diluted with an equal amount of water and undiluted Kreme O'Soy are commercial preparations of such a formula. The possible use of Cemac is suggested in the Infant Diet.

These diets, as discussed on page 145, may be modified according to the patient's definite or probable allergies and enlarged with additional foods according to recurring symptoms.

Elimination Diet in Infancy (Rowe)

Soy Bean Cereal-Free Formula (see directions, page 187).
Mull-Soy (Muller Laboratories, Baltimore, Md.).
Kreme O'Soy (Madison Foods, Madison College, Tenn.).
Sobee (Mead Johnson & Co.), 6 to 7 tablespoonfuls in 7 ounces of water boiled for three minutes.

Feedings of 5 to 8 ounces every four hours according to the infant's caloric requirements.   Two to 4 tablespoonfuls of cane sugar may be added to the daily amount of Mull-Soy, Kreme O'Soy or Soy Bean Formula. Similar amounts of Dextri-Maltose may be used if tolerated.

Sobee cooked with water for one-half hour may be used as a cereal, but the presence of arrowroot flour and olive oil in Sobee must be remembered.

If Soy-bean allergy or intolerance exists, Cemac (Mead Johnson & Co.) containing homogenized beef, vegetables, calcium, phosphorus, and iron may be tried.

For vitamin A, give Caritol in sesame oil, 8 to 10 drops daily.
For vitamin B_1 and B_2, give in feedings the contents of 2 B-complex capsules in feedings each day.
For vitamin C, give cevitamic acid, 50 mg. daily.
For vitamin D, give viosterol in sesame oil or Drisdol, 8 to 10 drops daily.

Adequate calcium and phosphorus are contained in the above soy bean preparations.

To the initial elimination diet, the following foods should also be added according to the infant's age, desire, digestive and allergic tolerance:

Grapefruit juice, sweetened, from the first to the third month.
Tomato juice may also be given if tolerated.
Puréed spinach, carrot, asparagus, beet, peas, string beans, lima beans, artichoke, tomato, from the third to the fourth month. (Trial of one or two at a time will evidence any allergic reactivity.)
Soft cooked white or sweet potato from the third to the fifth month.
Puréed pear, peach, apricot, or prune from the third to the sixth month.
Tapioca cooked with a little puréed fruit and sugar from the fourth to the sixth month.
Scraped or finely minced lamb or beef and also bacon from the eighth to the tenth month.

Butter substitutes such as Sesame Spread containing hydrogenated sesame oil, artificial color and flavor, and salt, or salted hydrogenated sesame oil may be used if desired.

Salt, cane or beet sugar, and sesame oil may also be used.

After relief is definite, the following foods may be added, one every five to ten days:

Orange, lemon, pineapple, apple, banana; cow's milk, evaporated or dried and later pasteurized; cream, butter; rice, corn, rye, wheat; chicken (no hens).

Eggs, chocolate, fish, and nuts should only be given to the child with atopic dermatitis during the second year.

Comments: The directions for the use of the elimination diet printed on page 155 should be read carefully. The use of clean utensils and dishes is important. As foods are added, their possible allergenic effect should be studied and, if symptoms recur, the causative foods should be eliminated (see page 145).

Elimination Diet After the First Year—Cereal–free (Rowe)

The amounts, ingredients, and preparation must vary according to the age, food allergies, food aversions, and digestive tolerance.

Foods Allowed

Soy Bean Cereal-Free Formula (see directions, page 187).

Mull-Soy (Muller Laboratories, 3156 Frederick Ave., Baltimore, Md.) (diluted with equal amount of water).

Kreme O'Soy (Madison Foods, Madison College, Tenn.) (undiluted).

Sobee (Mead Johnson & Co.), 6 tablespoonfuls in 7 ounces of water boiled for three minutes with added cane sugar or Dextri-Maltose as tolerated.

Tapioca	Lamb
White potato	Beef
Sweet potato	Bacon
Soy bean flour	Chicken (no hens)
Lima bean flour	
	Grapefruit
Spinach	Lemon
Chard	Peaches
Carrots	Pears
Beets	Apricots
Peas	Prunes
String beans	
Lima beans	Salt
Artichokes	Maple syrup (Log Cabin)
Asparagus	Sesame oil
Tomato	Sesame Spread (butter substitute)
	Soy bean oil

The Soy Bean Cereal-Free Formula, Mull-Soy or Kreme O'Soy may be used as such in a soup, or diluted as above, served hot or cold, sweetened if desired, and served throughout the day as a beverage. These contain all the important ingredients including calcium, phosphorus and protein found in milk. Sobee cooked for one-half hour may be used as a cereal if desired. Split pea purée, salted to taste and flavored with a little bacon may also be used as a drink or a soup.

BREAKFAST

Beverage:
　　Grapefruit juice, sweetened, *or*
　　Tomato juice (non-seasoned)
Cereal Substitute:
　　Tapioca cooked with pears, peaches, apricots or prunes, and sugar.
Bread:
　　Soy-lima or potato-lima bread or muffins made only according to recipes
　　　　in this book.(4a-4b; 5a-5b)
Butter Substitute:
　　Sesame Spread or salted, hydrogenated sesame oil if desired (see page 156).
Jams or Preserves:
　　Made from prescribed fruits and sugar, carrot marmalade, or tomato
　　　　preserves.(8)(9)
Meat:
　　Bacon, as such, if desired.

Soy Bean Cereal-Free Formula, Mull-Soy or Kreme O'Soy, 1 glassful.

LUNCH OR DINNER

Soup:
　　Beef or lamb broth—no pepper or onion—thickened with tapioca, potato
　　　　flour, or with a split pea purée. Vegetables listed in this diet may
　　　　be added, and soup may be salted to taste. (No canned soups
　　　　allowed.)
Meat:
　　Beef or lamb—chops, steak, hot or cold roast, cooked in their own fat
　　　　or in sesame oil.
　　Minced or ground beef or lamb.
　　Chicken—friers or broilers, (no hens). Rub and cook with sesame oil only.
Vegetables:
　　White or sweet potato, baked, boiled, or riced. May add Sesame Spread
　　　　or salt. Use no cow's milk or butter or any flour except potato, lima,
　　　　or soy flours.
　　Spinach, chard, carrots, beets, peas, string beans, lima beans, artichoke,
　　　　tomato, asparagus. (All cooked and possibly puréed. May add
　　　　Sesame Spread, sesame oil or soy bean oil, and salt.)
Bread:
　　Soy-lima or potato-lima bread or muffins as at breakfast with Sesame
　　　　Spread, jam or jelly allowed, carrot marmalade, or maple syrup.
　　　　(4)(5)(8)(9)
　　Tapioca cooked with pears, peaches, apricots and prunes, and sugar.(1)
　　Soy-lima or lima-potato cookies.(17)

Butter Substitute:
  As suggested for breakfast.
Fruit:
  Canned pears, peaches or apricots. Fresh peeled fruit may be ordered
  by physician.

Soy Bean Cereal-Free Formula, Mull-Soy, or Kreme O'Soy—1 glassful.

Instructions and Diet Suggestions

1. The use of elimination diets as summarized on page 155 and discussed in Chapter V must be accurately followed. Numbers in menus refer to recipes (page 237).

2. Give as much of all the foods with meals, and if desired between meals, as tolerated.

3. Weigh every two days. If weight loss occurs, give 1 to 2 teaspoonfuls of sesame oil between meals and more butter substitute or oil on the vegetables, more tapioca, potato, bread, cookies, jam, sugar, and maple syrup to increase calories.

4. Give meat or fowl twice a day and bacon once a day to assure protein balance.

5. Various puréed combinations of vegetables allowed in diet may be obtained. Libby, McNeil, Libby makes a homogenized one containing peas, carrots, spinach, and another with tomato, carrots, peas, etc. No drop or taste of any food not on the diet must be given. Foods must be served on clean plates, cooked in clean utensils. Do not stir child's food with a spoon that has touched other forbidden food like milk, egg, or butter without washing the spoon first.

6. If necessary to eat away from home, give prescribed plain meat, potato, vegetable, fruit or tomato juice with salt, canned fruit, sesame oils. The child's bread and cookies may be taken along.

7. If adequate Soy Bean Cereal-Free Formula, Mull-Soy, Kreme O'Soy or Sobee is not taken, then give 1 teaspoonful of dicalcium phosphate stirred up in $\frac{1}{3}$ glass of water or in divided doses on the food through the day.

8. Give cevitamic acid, 25 mg. once or twice daily, according to the amount of vitamin C in the fruits and vegetables taken.

9. Give Viosterol (Abbott) or Drisdol, 8 to 10 drops daily in food to assure adequate vitamin D. With adequate sun exposure, this may be omitted.

10. Give thiamin, 2 mg. daily, to assure adequate vitamin B_1.

11. After relief of allergy is definite, the following foods can be tried, one every five to seven days: rice, corn, orange, pineapple, apple, banana, cow's milk (at first canned or dried, and later pasteurized), butter, cream, wheat, eggs, fish, and other vegetables, fruits, and spices as relief continues. Any foods which produce immediate or delayed recurrences must be excluded.

Directions for Mixing the Soy Bean Formula (See next page)

All measurements are level and packed. Use standard tablespoon (Tbsp.) and teaspoon (tsp.) for measuring.

Soy Bean Cereal–free Formula (Rowe)

	Measure	Gm.	C., gm.	P., gm.	F., gm.	Cal.	Ca gm.	P gm.	Fe mg.	NaCl gm.
Soy bean flour*	11 Tbsp.	72.00	5.8	32.4	7.9	223	0.155	0.419	1.94	...
Soy bean oil	3 Tbsp.	30.00	...	...	30.0	270	....	....	...	...
Tapioca or arrowroot flour†	3 tsp.	10.00	10.0	...	...	40	....	....	...	...
Sugar	3 Tbsp.	32.00	32.0	...	...	128	....	....	...	...
Dicalcium phosphate	1¼ tsp.	4.30	...	...	...	..	1.000	0.774	...	...
NaCl	¼ tsp.	1.68	...	...	...	..	....	....	...	1.68
Water to make	32 oz.		47.8	32.4	37.9	661	1.155	1.193	1.94	1.68
This is the equivalent of	whole	milk.								
Whole milk	32 oz.	960	48.0	31.6	38.0	664	1.520	0.893	1.92	1.68

1. Put the soy bean oil in the top of a double boiler. Heat and add arrowroot or tapioca flour to make a smooth paste.

2. Add sugar, salt, dicalcium phosphate to 1 cup of hot water. Mix this with the soy bean flour to make a smooth paste, free of lumps. Add the extra water, to make 32 oz.

3. Add this mixture to No. 1 over the flame, stirring constantly. After the boiling point has been reached, cook for a few minutes. Replace kettle over the lower half of the double boiler. Cook twenty minutes.

* Staley's Soy Flour No. 1 (A. E. Staley Manufacturing Company, Decatur, Ill.) or Nutri Soy Flour No. 3 or 5 (Archer Daniels Midland Company, Minneapolis, Minn.) or similar processed soy bean flours make a smooth, non-precipitating emulsion. Raw soy bean flour produces an unsatisfactory product and its protein is precipitated as a "curd" when the calcium salts are added, especially by the more soluble calcium gluconate.

† Tapioca flour is less expensive than arrowroot flour and is obtainable at Irvine Company, 381 5th Street, Oakland, Calif., or at other baker's supply companies. If 4 teaspoonfuls of tapioca or arrowroot flour and 2⅔ tablespoonfuls of sugar are used, a thicker emulsion results with the same carbohydrate content.

(Carbohydrate, protein and fat values were obtained from Bridges, M.A.: Food and Beverage Analyses, Lea & Febiger, 1935, and the calcium, phosphorus and iron values from Bowes and Church: Food Values of Portions Commonly Used, Philadelphia Child Health Society, 1940, 311 S. Juniper Street, Philadelphia.)

REDUCTION DIETS FOR PATIENTS WITH DEFINITE OR POSSIBLE FOOD ALLERGIES

As noted previously many obese or over-weight patients are affected with symptoms due to definite or possible food allergies. For them, not only a low calorie diet with adequate protein content is necessary, but such a diet must be selected from the elimination diet chosen for diet trial by the physician.

Such diets, selected from foods in Elimination Diets 1 and 2, and also from Cereal-free Elimination Diets 1, 2 and 3, are detailed below.

Reduction Diets—Cereal-free Elimination Diets 1, 2 and 3 (Rowe)

Foods Allowed According to Menus Below

Tapioca
White potato
Sweet potato or yam

Lima bean-potato bread
Soy bean-lima bean bread
Soy bean-potato-tapioca bread

Lamb
Beef
Chicken
Bacon

Lettuce
Spinach
Chard
Carrots
Beets
Artichoke
Tomato
Squash
Asparagus
Peas
String beans
Lima beans

Lemon
Grapefruit
Pears
Pineapple
Peaches
Apricots

Salt
Sesame Spread
Gelatin, plain
Lime, lemon or pineapple
    flavored gelatin

White vinegar
Vanilla extract
Lemon extract

Royal baking powder
Baking soda
Cream of tartar
Saccharine

Suggested Menu—500 Calories

	Approximate amounts
Breakfast:	
Grapefruit juice	½ cup
Lunch:	
Clear lamb, beef or chicken broth (not canned)	1 cup
Lean lamb, beef or chicken—measure edible portion of cooked meat	¼ lb. scant
One vegetable from Group 1 (use lemon juice or white vinegar and salt on salads)	
One vegetable from Group 2	Amt. specified
One fruit from Group 3	Amt. specified
Lemonade with saccharine	
Dinner:	
Clear lamb, beef, or chicken broth (not canned)	1 cup
Lean lamb, beef, or chicken—measure edible portion of cooked meat	¼ lb. scant
Two vegetables from Group 1 (or one double portion) (use lemon juice or white vinegar and salt on salads)	Amt. specified
Two vegetables from Group 2	Amt. specified
One fruit from Group 3	Amt. specified

This menu contains approximately 500 calories

Carbohydrate	41 gm.	Ca	0.313 gm.
Protein	62 gm.	P	0.898 gm.
Fat	10 gm.	Fe	0.166 gm.

Suggested Menu—750 Calories

Approximate amounts

Breakfast:

Grapefruit juice	½ cup
Tapioca–soy bean–potato bread	1 slice 3 x 4 x ½″
Bacon—crisp	4 slices

Lunch:

Clear lamb, beef, or chicken broth (not canned)	1 cup
Lean lamb, beef or chicken—measure edible portion of cooked meat	2½ oz.
One vegetable from Group 1 (use lemon juice or white vinegar and salt on salads)	Amt. specified
One vegetable from Group 2	Amt. specified
One fruit from Group 3	Amt. specified
Lemonade with saccharine	

Dinner:

Clear lamb, beef or chicken broth (not canned)	1 cup
Lean meat—measure edible portion after cooking	¼ lb.
Two vegetables from Group 1 (or one double portion) (use lemon juice or white vinegar and salt on salads)	Amt. specified
Two vegetables from Group 2 (or one double portion)	Amt. specified
Tapioca–soy bean–potato bread	1 slice 3 x 4 x ½″
Sesame Spread	1 level tsp.
One fruit from Group 3	Amt. specified

This menu contains approximately 750 calories

Carbohydrate	53 gm.	Ca	0.337 gm.
Protein	69 gm.	P	0.935 gm.
Fat	29 gm.	Fe	0.015 gm.

Suggested Menu—1000 Calories

Breakfast:

Grapefruit juice	½ cup
Bacon—crisp	4 strips
Tapioca–soy bean–potato bread	1 slice 3 x 4 x ½″
Sesame Spread	1 level tsp.

Lunch:

Clear lamb, beef, or chicken broth (not canned)	1 cup
Lean lamb, beef, or chicken—measure edible portion after cooking	2½ oz.
One vegetable from Group 1 (use lemon juice or white vinegar and salt on salads)	Amt. specified
Two vegetables from Group 2	Amt. specified
One fruit from Group 3	Amt. specified
Lemonade with saccharine	

Dinner: *Approximate amounts*

    Clear lamb, beef, or chicken broth (not canned)   1 cup

    Lean lamb, beef or chicken   ¼ lb. scant

    White potato   1 med.

    Two vegetables from Group 1 (use lemon juice or white   Amt. specified
        vinegar and salt on salads)

    One vegetable from Group 2   Amt. specified

    Tapioca–soy bean–potato bread   1 slice 3 x 4 x ½″

    Sesame Spread   1 level tsp.

    One fruit from Group 3   Amt. specified

This menu contains approximately 1000 calories

Carbohydrate	103 gm.	Ca	0.350 gm.
Protein	72 gm.	P	0.988 gm.
Fat	34 gm.	Fe	0.016 gm.

Vegetables and Fruits
(Measured after cooking)

Group 1:

    Spinach—fresh, cooked or canned   ½ cup

    Chard—cooked   ⅓ cup

    Asparagus—cooked   6 stalks

    Squash—cooked   ¼ cup

    Lettuce—4 large leaves or ⅓ med. head

Group 2:

    Carrots—cooked   ½ cup

    Beets—cooked   ⅓ cup

    Artichoke—fresh cooked   1 medium

    Artichoke—canned   4 small hearts

    Tomato—fresh   1 med.

    Tomato—canned   ½ cup

    Tomato—juice   ½ cup

    Squash—cooked   ¾ cup

    Green peas—cooked   ¼ cup

    String beans—cooked   ⅔ cup

    Green lima beans—cooked   2 Tbsp.

Group 3:

    Grapefruit—fresh   ½ small 3½″ diam.

    Grapefruit—canned without sugar   ½ cup

    Grapefruit—juice canned without sugar   ½ cup

    Pears—fresh   1 small

    Pears—canned in water   2 halves

    Pineapple—fresh, diced   ½ cup

    Pineapple—canned in water   1 small slice

    Pineapple—juice, not sweetened   ¼ cup

    Peaches—fresh   1 small

    Peaches—canned in water   2 halves

    Apricots—fresh   2 whole

    Apricots—canned in water   2 whole

    Gelatin—lemon, lime or pineapple   4 level Tbsp.

    D-Zerta—lemon or lime, may be used as desired

Comments: The suggestions and directions about the preparation of the elimination diets as summarized on pages 148 and 155 are most necessary to remember. Broths (not canned) should be made from plain meats, with no condiments, pastes, or added ingredients except salt and prescribed vegetables. Only fresh or water packed specified fruits permitted. No trace of any food not included in the elimination diet is allowable. Recipes for bakery products are on page 237.

To assure calcium balance, 3 teaspoonfuls of calcium gluconate or 1 teaspoonful of calcium carbonate should be taken with water daily. Viosterol in sesame oil, 12 to 15 drops, is necessary if skin exposure to the sun or ultra-violet light is not available. Additional thiamin and cevitamic acid therapy is necessary, especially with low calorie diets. (See page 146.)

Reduction Diets—Elimination Diets 1 and 2 (Rowe)

Foods Allowed According to Menus Below

Rice	Lettuce
Corn	Chard
Rye	Spinach
Tapioca	Carrots
Sweet potato or yam	Beets
	Squash
Rice Biscuit	Asparagus
Rice bread	Artichoke
Corn pone	
Corn-rye muffins	Saccharine
Rye bread	Salt
Ry-Krisp	Sesame Spread
	Gelatin, plain
Lemon	Lime, lemon or pineapple
Grapefruit	flavored gelatin
Pears	White vinegar
Pineapple	
Peaches	Vanilla extract
Apricots	Lemon extract
Prunes	Royal baking powder
	Baking soda
Lamb	Cream of tartar
Chicken (no hens)	
Bacon	

Suggested Menu—500 Calories

	Approximate amounts
Breakfast:	
Grapefruit juice	½ cup
Lunch:	
Clear lamb or chicken broth (not canned)	1 cup
Lean lamb or chicken—measure only edible portion of cooked meat	¼ lb.
One vegetable from Group 1 (use lemon juice or white vinegar on salad)	Amt. specified

Suggested Menu—500 Calories—(Continued)

	Approximate amounts
Lunch:	
One vegetable from Group 2	Amt. specified
One fruit from Group 3	Amt. specified
Lemonade with saccharine	
Dinner:	
Clear lamb or chicken broth (not canned)	1 cup
Lean lamb or chicken—measure only edible portion of cooked meat	$\frac{1}{4}$ lb.
Two vegetables from Group 1 or one double portion (use lemon juice or white vinegar on salad)	Amt. specified
Two vegetables from Group 2 or one double portion	Amt. specified
One fruit from Group 3	Amt. specified
Lemonade with saccharine	

This menu contains approximately 500 calories

Carbohydrate	46 gm.	Ca	0.315 gm.
Protein	60 gm.	P	0.900 gm.
Fat	9 gm.	Fe	0.017 gm.

Suggested Menu—750 Calories

	Approximate amounts
Breakfast:	
Grapefruit juice	$\frac{1}{2}$ cup
Ry-Krisp	2 wafers
Bacon—crisp	4 slices
Lunch:	
Clear lamb or chicken broth (not canned)	1 cup
Lean lamb or chicken—measure only edible portion of cooked meat	$\frac{1}{4}$ lb.
One vegetable from Group 1 (use lemon juice or white vinegar and salt on salads)	Amt. specified
One vegetable from Group 2	Amt. specified
Ry-Krisp	2 wafers
One fruit from Group 3	Amt. specified
Lemonade with saccharine.	

	Approximate amounts
Dinner:	
Clear lamb or chicken broth (not canned)	$\frac{1}{4}$ cup
Lean lamb or chicken—measure only edible portion of cooked meat	$\frac{1}{4}$ lb.
Two vegetables from Group 1 or one double portion (use lemon juice or white vinegar and salt on salads)	Amt. specified
Two vegetables from Group 2 or one double portion	Amt. specified
Ry-Krisp	2 wafers
One fruit from Group 3	Amt. specified
Lemonade with saccharine	

This menu contains approximately 750 calories.

Carbohydrate	70 gm.	Ca	0.340 gm.
Protein	75 gm.	P	0.926 gm.
Fat	19 gm.	Fe	0.016 gm.

Suggested Menu—1,000 Calories

	Approximate amounts
Breakfast:	
Grapefruit juice	½ cup
Ry-Krisp	2 wafers
Bacon—crisp	4 slices
Lunch:	
Clear lamb or chicken broth (not canned)	1 cup
Lean lamb or chicken—measure only edible portion of cooked meat	¼ lb.
One vegetable from Group 1 (use lemon juice or white vinegar and salt on salads)	Amt. specified
Two vegetables from Group 2 or one double portion	Amt. specified
Ry-Krisp	2 wafers
Sesame Spread	1 level tsp.
One fruit from Group 3	Amt. specified
Lemonade with saccharine	
Dinner:	
Clear lamb or chicken broth	1 cup
Lean lamb or chicken—measure only edible portion of cooked meat	¼ lb.
Corn *or*	1 med. ear or ½ cup
Rice—steamed	1 heap. Tbsp.
Two vegetables from Group 1 or one double portion (use lemon juice or white vinegar and salt on salads)	Amt. specified
One vegetable from Group 2	Amt. specified
Ry-Krisp	1 wafer
Sesame Spread	1 level Tbsp.
One fruit from Group 3	Amt. specified
Lemonade with saccharine	

This menu contains approximately 1000 calories.

Carbohydrate	89 gm.	Ca	0.380 gm.
Protein	76 gm.	P	1.000 gm.
Fat	38 gm.	Fe	0.017 gm.

Vegetables and Fruits
(Measured after cooking)

Group 1:	Amounts
Spinach—fresh cooked or canned	½ cup
Chard—cooked	⅓ cup
Asparagus—cooked	6 stalks
Squash—cooked	¼ cup
Lettuce	4 large leaves or ⅓ med. head

13

Vegetables and Fruits—(Continued)

(Measured after cooking)

Group 2:	*Amounts*
Carrots—cooked	½ cup
Beets—cooked	⅓ cup
Artichoke—fresh cooked	1 medium
Artichoke—canned	4 small hearts
Squash—cooked	¾ cup
Group 3:	
Grapefruit—fresh	½ small 3½″ diam.
Grapefruit—canned without sugar	½ cup
Grapefruit juice—canned without sugar	½ cup
Pears—fresh	1 small
Pears—canned in water	2 halves
Pineapple—fresh, diced	½ cup
Pineapple—canned in water	1 small slice
Pineapple juice—not sweetened	¼ cup
Peaches—fresh	1 small
Peaches—canned in water	2 halves
Apricots—fresh	2 whole
Apricots—canned in water	2 whole
Gelatin—lemon, lime or pineapple flavored	4 level Tbsp.
D-Zerta—lemon or lime—may be used as desired	

Comments: Similar diets containing the same amounts of carbohydrate, protein and fat may be arranged from other foods on Elimination Diets 1 and 2. (See page 161.)

The suggestions and directions about the preparation of the elimination diets as summarized on pages 148 and 155 are most necessary to remember. Broths (not canned) should be made from plain meats, salted to taste, and no condiments, pastes or added ingredients except prescribed vegetables should be used. No trace of any food not included in these elimination diets is allowable.

DIABETIC DIETS SELECTED FROM FOODS IN THE ELIMINATION DIETS

As discussed on page 153, various diabetic patients either suffer from definite and obvious food allergies or have symptoms which require a careful study of possible food allergy. The following diets are models on which the diet of any diabetic can be formulated so that it contains those foods in the elimination diet chosen by the physician for the study of possible food allergy in the patient.

The physician can order the following diet and the dietitian or his office assistant can prepare menus accordingly.

Diabetic Diet from Cereal-free Elimination Diets 1, 2 and 3 (Rowe)

(Carbohydrate 70 gm., protein 25 gm., fat 40 gm. per meal.
Calories per day, 2220.)

Suggested Menu

BREAKFAST (1)

	Amount	Wt. in gm.	Carb.	Prot.	Fat
Pineapple juice, unsweetened	½ cup	120	16	..	..
Soy bean tapioca bread	2 slices	..	17.4	6	6.6
Sesame Spread	2 Tbsp.	20	..	..	16
Tapioca cooked with dried	2 Tbsp. dry wt.	20	17	..	..
Prunes and 1 cup water	3 med.	70	20	..	..
Lean meat patty	2 oz. cooked wt.	60	..	16	5
Bacon—medium	3 strips	15	..	4.5	12
	Total		70.4	26.5	39.6

BREAKFAST (2)

	Amount	Wt. in gm.	Carb.	Prot.	Fat
Grapefruit juice	½ cup	120	11.5	0.5	..
Apricots, fresh or water packed	2 whole	100	10	1	..
Soy bean tapioca bread	2 slices	..	17.4	6	6.6
Sesame Spread	2 Tbsp.	20	..	..	16
Potatoes, cold boiled, browned	1 med.	150	32	3.8	..
in sesame oil	1 Tbsp.	14	..	..	14
Lean beef or lamb	1⅔ oz. cooked wt.	52	..	14	4
	Total		70.9	25.3	40.6

LUNCH

	Amount	Wt. in gm.	Carb.	Prot.	Fat
Lean beef, cooked E.P.	1½ oz.	42	..	11.5	2.3
Green lima beans	½ cup	75	17.6	5.6	0.6
White potato, boiled	1 med.	150	31.4	3.8	..
Tomato served with	1 small	125	4.1	1.1	..
Sesame oil and	1 Tbsp.	14	..	..	14.0
White vinegar or lemon juice					
Soy bean tapioca bread	1 slice	..	8.7	3.0	3.3
Sesame Spread	2½ Tbsp.	25	..	..	20.0
Pears, fresh or water packed	1 small	100	8.3	..	..
	Total		70.1	25.0	40.2

DINNER

	Amount	Wt. in gm.	Carb.	Prot.	Fat
Clear chicken, beef or lamb broth (not canned)					
Tomato juice	½ cup	120	4.3	1.2	..
Lean lamb or chicken, E.P.	1½ oz.	45	..	12.0	2.6
String beans	⅔ cup	130	4.5	1.3	..
White potato, baked	1 med.	150	38.1	4.6	..
Asparagus salad	6 stalks	85	1.4	2.1	..
Sesame oil	1 Tbsp.	14	..	..	14.0
White vinegar or lemon juice					
Soy bean tapioca bread	1 slice	..	8.7	3.0	3.3
Sesame Spread	2½ Tbsp.	25	..	..	20.0
Peaches, fresh or water packed	1 med.	150	13.2	0.8	..
	Total		70.3	25.0	39.9

Comments: Other foods in Cereal-free Elimination Diets 1, 2 and 3, in amounts containing the required grams of carbohydrate, protein and fat may be substituted for those in the above menu. The preparation of this elimination type of diabetic diet and the use of calcium and additional vitamins should follow the suggestions on pages 146 and 155.

As with other elimination diets, their use as discussed on page 155 must be carefully read and followed. Insulin therapy, of course, as indicated by the diabetes must be given. Similar diets satisfying other food allowances for diabetic patients and containing other foods for the special allergic problem of the patient can be prepared.

Diabetic Diet from Elimination Diets 1 and 2 (Rowe)

(Carbohydrate 70 gm., protein 25 gm., fat 40 gm. per meal.
Calories per day, 2220.)

Suggested Menu

BREAKFAST

	Amount	Wt. in gm.	Carb.	Prot.	Fat
Grapefruit juice	⅔ cup	135	13.0	0.6	..
Peaches cooked with juice or water packed—no sugar added . .	1 med.	150	13.0	0.8	..
Rice or corn flakes	1 cup	30	26.0	2.0	..
Corn and rice muffins with	1 muffin	..	18.0	1.7	7.6
Sesame Spread	2 Tbsp.	20	..	..	16.0
Lamb patties, lean lamb cooked, E.P.	2 oz.	60	..	16.0	5.0
Bacon, medium	3 strips	10	..	4.5	12.0
		Total	70.1	24.4	40.0

LUNCH

	Amount	Wt. in gm.	Carb.	Prot.	Fat
Lamb chops or roast, fat removed, cooked, E.P.	2 oz.	60	..	18.0	5.0
Steamed rice	½ cup	100	22.5	2.3	1.0
Steamed carrots	¾ cup	100	6.6	1.0	..
Asparagus salad with dressing of	8 stalks	100	2.3	1.5	..
Sesame oil and	1 Tbsp.	14	..	..	14.0
Lemon juice or white vinegar					
Ry-Krisp	2	12	7.4	1.6	..
Sesame Spread	2½ Tbsp.	25	..	..	20.0
Apricots, fresh or water packed .	3 whole	140	15.4	..	..
Pineapple juice, unsweetened. .	½ cup	120	15.9	..	..
		Total	70.1	24.4	40.0

DINNER

	Amount	Wt. in gm.	Carb.	Prot.	Fat
Clear lamb or chicken broth					
Grapefruit—fresh	½—4″ diam.	100	9.8	0.5	..
Chicken, visible fat removed, cooked, E.P.	2 oz.	65	..	18.0	8.0
Sweet potato, baked	½ large	100	32.0	2.0	..
Spinach	½ cup	100	0.8	2.0	..
Artichoke salad with White vinegar and	1 large globe or 5 small hearts, canned	125	5.5	1.0	..
Sesame oil	1 Tbsp.	14	..	..	14.0
Rye bread—100%	1 slice	25	13.0	2.0	..
Sesame Spread	2¼ Tbsp.	22	..	..	18.0
Pineapple, fresh diced or	⅔ cup	100	10.0	..	..
Water packed	1 slice	75	10.0	..	.
		Total	71.1	25.5	40.0

Other foods in Elimination Diets 1 and 2 in amounts containing the required grams of carbohydrate, protein and fat may be substituted for those in the above menu. The preparation of this elimination type of diabetic diet and the use of calcium and additional vitamins should follow the suggestions on pages 146 and 155.

As with other elimination diets, their use as discussed on page 155 must be carefully read and followed. Insulin therapy, of course, as indicated by the diabetes must be given. Similar diets satisfying other food allowances for diabetic patients and containing other foods for the special allergic problem of the patient can be prepared.

THE WHEAT-FREE DIET

The wheat-free diet is indicated when a definite allergy to wheat exists. Clinical allergy, as in all food allergy, may occur without a positive skin reaction. It is unusual to be allergic to wheat alone. Sensitizations to other foods, usually to some of the important ones, including milk, egg, rice, corn, fish, orange, apple, banana, etc., may exist along with wheat allergy. Therefore, especially where food allergy is suspected, it is better to use the elimination diets rather than a wheat-free diet during a period of diagnostic study of possible food allergy.

However, when wheat alone is to be excluded from the diet, the following facts must be remembered. Every trace of wheat must be excluded when marked allergy exists. The toasting or super-heating of wheat bread or other wheat products does not denaturize the allergen sufficiently to prevent reactions in the very allergic individual. Bakery products must be made at home or by supervised or trusted bakers with flours which are wheat-free. Ordinary rye and most pumpernickel bread contains varying amounts of wheat flour. Commercial rice, corn, soy, lima, and potato breads all contain wheat or gluten wheat flours. Most so-called self-rising flours, pancake and cake flours, health grains and brans contain wheat. Grapenuts, Pep, and many other breakfast foods, as listed on page 232, contain wheat. Today, the content of all food products of the above types are listed on the labels. However, changes may occur before labels are changed. Macaroni, vermicelli, noodles, so-called pastes, and most tamales, enchilades, and other so-called Spanish or Mexican foods, especially those sold commercially, contain wheat and, at times, milk or egg. Vitavose and other vitamin products may contain wheat germ. Many soups have had pastes cooked in them or are thickened with wheat flour. These are only a few possibilities of the use of wheat in various foods and recipes.

The wheat-free diet, therefore, demands dependable wheat-*free* breads, cookies, cakes, and other bakery products. Recipes are available on pages 237 to 257. Ry-Krisp is a desirable wheat-free cracker. Some rye crisps are dusted with wheat flour. Various Mexican foods, made with corn meal are desirable, but frequently wheat flour is included. Corn crisps, potato chips, rice-corn muffins, corn pone, and various corn, rice, barley, oats, and rye dry and cooked cereal products are useful. Various flours, including potato, cassava, banana, chestnut, almond, pea, bean, peanut, lima, soy, poya, sweet potato, pumpkin, and others are available for wheat-free diets.

THE EGG-FREE DIET

The egg-free diet demands a most careful selection of foods. As a trial diet, it is unusually inadvisable since few patients are only sensitive to egg. However, egg may finally prove after a period of trial dieting, to be the one important food to which allergy exists. When egg allergy is present, it is practically always necessary to exclude the albumen and the yolk, since it is difficult to entirely separate the yolk from all albumen.

Egg is used in practically all ice cream, sherbets, and water ices, cakes, cookies, many French toasts, puddings, desserts, mayonnaise, and other sauces, and salad dressings. Macaroni, spaghetti, noodles, batters, prepared meats, some sausages, beef juices, and meat jellies contain egg. It is in many candies and bar confections, and certain marshmallows. Bread, buns, and pretzels may be rubbed or sprayed with egg to produce a sheen or crust. Rumford's baking powder, Ovaltine, Ovomalt, and Cocamalt contain egg. Soups, coffee, and certain wines may be cleared with egg white. Some pharmaceutical products and emulsions contain some egg. Thus, special recipes must be used in the home and by bakers for patients on egg-free diets.

Eggs of various birds contain similar allergens and many patients who are sensitive to hen's egg are also allergic to duck, goose, or turkey eggs. Some mildly allergic patients can tolerate the denaturized hard boiled egg.

Some patients are so sensitive to egg that they cannot handle egg or have eggs on the table or eat food kept in a refrigerator in which eggs are present. Such patients should not be kissed by a person who has just eaten egg because of residual amounts on the lips. Some egg-sensitive patients, moreover, are also sensitive to chicken meat. This is especially true of hen meat since a moderate amount of egg allergen may get onto the hen during the cleaning of the bird.

THE MILK-FREE DIET

Certain patients may be allergic only to milk. Its exclusion from the diet necessitates the elimination of every trace of milk in the very allergic patient. In infancy, a milk substitute such as the soy bean preparations becomes necessary as discussed on pages 183 to 187.

Sobee, as originated by Hill, and prepared by Mead Johnson & Co., is a dry powder of the following formula:

	Per cent		Per cent
Soy bean flour	61	Dextri-Maltose	6
Olive oil	19	Dicalcium phosphate	4
Arrowroot starch	9	Sodium chloride	1

When 6 to 7 tablespoonfuls are added to 7 ounces of water, brought to a boil and cooled, and sugar is added according to the physician's order, a palatable, easily digested milk substitute is made. Its approximate content follows:

	Per cent		Per cent
Fat	2.8	Salts	1.0
Protein	4.2	Carbohydrates	4.1

As stated on page 184, Sobee also can be cooked with water as a mush.

Fluid preparations similar to Sobee are available. Mull-Soy when diluted with an equal amount of water and Kreme O'Soy used undiluted, contain about the same constituents as cow's milk.

A soy bean emulsion which is quite acceptable can be made inexpensively by the detailed directions found on page 187. The protein, calcium and calorie content as indicated is identical to that of cow's milk.

For those infants who can not take soy bean, Cemac, as prepared by Mead Johnson & Co. is available. This was proposed by Cohen in 1933 similar to a formula the writer published in 1931. (See page 257.) Recently, homogenized liquid lamb, beef and liver have been prepared with which individualized formulæ similar to Cemac may be made at home according to the child's nutritional demands, possible allergies and the physician's orders.

In children and adults, the milk-free diet demands most careful scrutiny of all ingested mixed foods to prevent the ingestion of a trace of any milk or its products. It must be remembered that practically all commercial breads, cakes, and most cookies and other bakery products, contain milk, often in powdered form or butter. The presence of milk in many canned soups, in Ovaltine, Cocamalt, milk chocolate, malted milk, many candies, ice cream, practically all sherbets and commercial ices, must be remembered. Many patients fail to realize that cream contains from 60 to 85 per cent milk, and that butter contains .5 to 1.5 per cent milk solids. Moreover, oleomargarines of all types, including Nucoa, contain from 1.5 to 2 per cent milk solids. Many pies, breads, and other bakery products are sprayed with milk. Milk or butter is used in mashed potato, souffles, many gravies, sauces, puddings, custards, and various desserts.

Some patients are allergic to the milk of one animal and not of another. The lactalbumins of milks of different animals are dissimilar. Thus, goat's milk can be tolerated by some infants and children who are sensitive to the lactalbumen of cow's milk. The caseins of the milks of different animals seem identical and allergy thereto explains sensitization to milks of several animals. In Europe, the milks of the ass, mare, and ewe are used.

The denaturization of milk by heat has been discussed on page 60. As there stated, some mildly milk-sensitive patients can tolerate heated and canned milk. However, if milk allergy is suspected, every trace of milk in all forms should be eliminated from the diet until symptoms are definitely controlled. This, of course, has been done in the elimination diets.

The kind of milk in various cheeses has been discussed on page 70. Other ingredients, including fungi of varying types in cheeses must be remembered.

The milk-free diet, together with practically every other diet, needs supplemental vitamin D, especially during the Fall to Spring months. The ways in which this may be taken are discussed on page 146. *It is the writer's opinion that it is usually better to use the elimination diets when milk is to be excluded from the diet.* As stated above, milk and its products enter into so many bakery products and other foods that it is usually very difficult for the patient to have foods prepared and cooked so that every trace of milk is excluded. The elimination diets, on the other hand, are milk-free, and in addition, they exclude many other foods which with varying frequencies produce food allergy in patients. After symptoms are relieved, the various foods can be added.*

ADDITION OF FOODS TO THE DIET

As important foods are added to the elimination diet, the physician must discuss the various ways in which this may be done. The addition of milk and egg is usually easy for the patient. The addition of wheat needs special discussion, and rice and corn, particularly, before milk and eggs are added, need specific instructions. *To conserve the physician's time, and to furnish the patient with explicit directions, the following suggestions have been prepared.*

Addition of Wheat to the Elimination Diet.—Wheat alone is contained in Shredded Wheat, Farina, Cream of Wheat, Wheatina, and other cereal products on page 232 and various crackers as indicated in the listed ingredients on the labels.

Wheat flour, either the refined, whole wheat, graham, or gluten may be used. The addition of such flour, especially gluten flour because of the gliadin content (see page 62) to recipes for the various wheat, milk, and egg-free bakery products in this volume adds greatly to lightness and palatability.

When wheat is added, white or other wheat bread and various bakery products containing wheat are not necessarily allowed. All of these contain various ingredients which may not be in the patient's diet. The fact that milk, egg, various oils or shortenings and other cereal grains are included must be remembered. White bread practically always contains milk, at times egg or some other flour especially to prevent sticking to pans. Also the use of various shortenings containing cottonseed and other oils or fats must be remembered.

Addition of Rice.—Boiled rice served hot with cane sugar or maple syrup or served as such in place of potatoes or as cereal.

* Hill has reported maintenance of protein nutrition with amino-acids in milk sensitive infants, J. A. M. A., **116**, 2135, 1941.

Cold boiled rice fried in sesame oil or other specified oil served with maple syrup or sugar, or any of the fruit juices allowed on the diet.

Rice cooked with a small amount of pears, peaches, or apricots and sugar as a pudding.

Rice flakes and Rice Krispies served with any of the fruit juices allowed on the diet and sugar.

Puffed Rice served with fruit juices and sugar or made into candy according to the recipe on page 248.

Brown rice or wild rice can also be used, cooked alone or in any of the ways noted above. Cream of Rice, a packaged cereal, cannot be used since it contains powdered milk.

If corn or rye has been added to the diet, bread, muffins, and cookies can be made by combining corn or rye flour with rice flour according to the recipes on page 245. Rice bread may also be made (page 246).

Addition of Corn.—Canned corn (cream style), whole kernel, or on the cob, fresh or canned. No butter or other seasonings which are not allowed on the diet should be used. Sesame butter substitute (see page 156) may be used if desired.

Cornmeal may be cooked with water and a pinch of salt to make a mush. This may be served hot with fruit juices and sugar or maple syrup. The cold cornmeal mush may be fried in sesame oil and served with maple syrup. Polenta, a coarse cornmeal, may be cooked as above.

Corn flakes served with any of the fruit juices allowed on the diet and sugar.

Canned hominy can be fried in sesame oil and served with maple syrup.

Mazola oil may be used in cooking if desired.

Cornstarch may be used in cooking and fruit cornstarch pudding can be made according to the recipe on page 248.

Corn syrup such as Karo may be used in the candy recipes, in cooking, and as a substitute for maple syrup.

Corn pone may be made according to the recipe on page 245.

If rice or rye have been added to the diet, bread, muffins, and cookies can be made by combining rice or rye flour with cornmeal, according to the recipes on pages 245 and 246.

CHAPTER VI

APPENDIX

VITAMINS

Their Characteristics, Distribution and Requirements

Vitamin A is fat soluble and is not destroyed by freezing or boiling or by the high temperatures of canning, provided oxidation is prevented. It may rapidly diminish after defrosting. Drying of foods may decrease this vitamin because of oxidation. Mineral oil by mouth, taken for constipation, absorbs Vitamin A and its precursor from the food. If taken only one to two times a day, well after meals, such absorption is not serious.

Vitamin A, in its precursor, the yellow pigment, carotene, usually occurs with chlorophyll in green leaves. The white or light parts of the plant have little of this vitamin. The yellow and green leaf vegetables and carrots, sweet potatoes, and lettuce, chard, and parsley are rich in Vitamin A. Apricots contain more than other fruits. The large amount of Vitamin A in fish oils comes from the minute marine plants which are eaten by small fish which, in turn, are eaten by larger fish such as the cod and halibut. One U.S.P. unit is contained in .3 microgram of crystalline vitamin. Deficiency of Vitamin A, according to McLester, disturbs the structural integrity of epithelial cells.

In patients allergic to vegetables and fruits, the daily requirement of Vitamin A as listed below, must be assured. This can be computed from the average vitamin content of foods in recent published tables.*

Vitamin B, known as thiamin, has been synthesized in crystalline form. It occurs in varying amounts in many plant and animal foods, especially in the germ or outer covering of cereal grains and seeds, in milk, eggs, liver, yeast, and fruits and vegetables. It is not broken down easily by cooking except in an alkaline medium. It is water soluble so that vegetables should be cooked in as little water as is possible.

It seems that 1 or 2 mg. of thiamin are sufficient for health

---

* The latest table of vitamins A and D in international units, thiamin and riboflavin in micrograms and ascorbic acid in milligrams can be obtained from Dr. E. Booher, U. S. Department of Agriculture, Bureau of Home Economics, Washington, D. C.

but that 10 or more mg. daily are necessary when a deficiency state has arisen from a long standing lack of this vitamin. Williams and Spies have estimated that 1 mg. of thiamin equals approximately 250 International units of B. The approximate amounts of Vitamin B_1 in foods are in recent tables.

Vitamin G or riboflavin (B_2) is water soluble and is a greenish yellow substance of the flavin group. It influences the oxidation in the cell and the general health of the body. Its lack seems to cause lesions on lips and angles of the mouth known as cheilitis. Man apparently requires 2 to 3 mg. of riboflavin a day. One Sherman-Bourquin unit of Vitamin G is supplied by 3 to 5 micrograms of riboflavin. One milligram thus contains from 200 to 300 units. Foods containing the most riboflavin are: milk, eggs, liver, and the green leaf vegetables. Liver contains about fifteen times as much as meat.

Nicotinic Acid is one of the vitamins in the so-called B complex. Its curative action in pellagra has been demonstrated by investigations, especially of Elvehjem, Spies, and their collaborators. It is found in yeast, liver, lean meats, and milk. For moderate deficiencies, 50 to 100 mg. are given three times a day, either by mouth or parenterally in solution. Large doses up to 1000 mg. a day may be desirable.

Vitamin H (B_6) is called the antidermatitic factor of the B complex. It is synthesized as a pyridine base. Its lack leads to cessation of growth, an erythedemic dermatosis, and general debility. Certain patients with pellagra and beriberi with central nervous system manifestations require 50 mg. of this vitamin daily, as well as nicotinic acid, thiamin, and riboflavin, according to Spies.

Vitamin C (ascorbic or cevitamic acid) controls the formation of the intercellular reticulum and bands of collagen in tissue cells. Its lack in the diet results in scurvy associated with increased capillary fragility, anemia, weakness, and reduced resistance to infection. It is prescribed in its synthetic form. The international unit is .05 mg.

Vitamin C is decreased in varying degrees by drying, canning, cooking, freezing, or storing of foods. Contact with metal, exposure to heat, light, air, and especially to oxidation, is detrimental. Canned products, protected only against oxidation, show a slight decrease in Vitamin C.

Increased amounts are required during infections and when a deficiency has existed. The daily requirements of Vitamin C are listed below.

The approximate amounts of cevitamic acid (Vitamin C) in 100 gram amounts of various fruits and vegetables are listed in recent tables (see page 203). The content varies as much as 50 per cent with the type of soil and weather conditions.

Vitamin D is fat soluble and controls the concentration of the calcium and phosphate ions in the blood so that proper bone calcification occurs. Deficiency of this vitamin produces rickets and associated symptoms. Irradiation of cereals, meat, milk, eggs, fats, oils, various vegetables, and many other foods, and especially the sterol of ergot called ergosterol produces mainly a crystalline substance called calciferol which is probably pure Vitamin D.

Several forms of Vitamin D are known. Activated ergosterol obtained chiefly from irradiation of yeast is in viosterol and in the milk of cows which have been fed irradiated yeast. Activated 7-dehydrocholesterol results from the action of sunlight and other ultra-violet rays upon animal fats. It is present in irradiated milk and is the main form of Vitamin D in antirachitic fish oils. Both these forms of Vitamin D seem of equal therapeutic potency in man. Sunlight or ultra-violet rays on the skin also convert the provitamin in the oily secretions into Vitamin D which is absorbed by the blood. One U.S.P. or International unit is the activity of .025 microgram of crystalline Vitamin D. Only .25 gram is in a barrel of ordinary cod liver oil.

Vitamin D does not occur in many foods. Fish, especially those containing body oil such as salmon, sardines, and herring, contain moderate amounts. The oils of the livers of blue fin tuna especially, of sword fish, yellow fin tuna, and black sea bass contain large amounts. The oils of the livers of many rock fish, cod, halibut, salmon, and to a lesser extent of many other fish, contain decreasing amounts of Vitamin D. Cow's milk, especially during the summer, contains moderate amounts of this vitamin. Eggs also contain a fair quantity.

Cod liver and other fish oils, therefore, vary in their content of Vitamin D. This is especially true when they are fortified with viosterol. The content of each preparation must be determined by the label. The requirements for Vitamin D are noted below. The requirement of the adult is in question. Considerable amounts are manufactured by the action of sunlight on the skin.

Vitamin E was discovered and isolated in its pure form by Evans and Bishop. Its lack results in failure of placental and foetal development and degeneration in the male and female germ cells. Muscular dystrophies in man, sterility and habitual abortion may be due at times to a deficiency of Vitamin E. It is widely distributed in foods, especially in milk, butter, grains, and vegetables. It is stable at high temperatures and in light.

Vitamin K maintains the prothrombin level in the blood and thus the clotting time. Its absorption is aided by bile in the intestine. The bleeding of obstructive jaundice is benefited by administration of this vitamin. It is especially abundant in alfalfa and is found along with Vitamin C in other foods.

DAILY NUTRITIONAL REQUIREMENTS

Vitamins

Vitamin A:
Infants . . . . 6,000–10,000 units
Children . . . . 8,000–12,000 units
Adults . . . . 6,000– 9,000 units
Vitamin B$_1$:
All ages . . . . 1–3 mg.
Vitamin B$_2$:
All ages . . . . 1–3 mg.
Vitamin C:
Infants . . . . 50 mg.
Children . . . . 50–100 mg.
Adults . . . . 50–100 mg.
Vitamin D:
Infancy, Childhood and Adolescence . . . 300–400 units
Pregnancy . . . . 800 units
Adults . . . . 300–500 units

(Units are International)

Calories

(Total requirements daily—Sansum, Hare and Bowden)*

CHILDREN

Age	Calories per 24 hrs.
1½–2 years	1000–1200
2–4 years	1200–1400
4–6 years	1400–1600
6–8 years	1600–1800
8–10 years	1800–2000
10–12 years	2000–2200
Adolescent youth	2200–5500

ADULTS

	Men	Women
Resting	1200–1500	1000–1200
Very light work	1500–2000	1500–1800
Light work	2000–2500	1800–2200
Moderately heavy work	2500–3000	2200–2500
Heavy work	3000–3500	2500–3000
Hard manual labor	3500–4000	

* From Normal Diet and Healthful Living, Sansum, W. D., Hare, R. A., and Bowden, D., The Macmillan Company, 1936.

MAINTENANCE OF WEIGHT

The elimination diets require a change in eating habits. If it is important to maintain or increase weight, the physician must tell the patient to take adequate amounts of the starches, bakery products, sugar, jams and jellies, butter substitute and oils on the diet so that adequate calories will be ingested. It is usually necessary to discuss all the various foods which contain calories with the patient. The patient may well keep the following suggestions at hand so that undesirable weight loss will not occur.

The Maintaining or Increasing of Weight.—1. You should weigh every other day, and if undesirable weight loss occurs, foods allowed in the diet which are rich in calories should be taken.

2. You should take plenty of the specified oils on salads and vegetables. In addition, 1 to 6 teaspoonsfuls of such oil are to be taken after every meal. This amount varies according to your age and your digestive tolerance.

3. You should eat plenty of the bread, cookies, muffins, and other bakery products made according to the special recipes or prepared by bakers designated by your physician. More of these can be taken if plenty of jam, jelly, and maple syrup are used on them.

4. A butter substitute made of a prescribed fat such as sesame oil (see page 156) entirely free of milk products may be used in good amounts.

5. Plenty of jam and jelly should be used in breads and cookies allowed in the diet. Specified fruits on the diet should be used for jams and jellies.

6. Plenty of sugar should be used in fruit drinks and in desserts. Tapioca should be cooked with fruit and plenty of sugar.

7. Log Cabin or plain maple syrup may also be used on any foods in your diet in order to increase your caloric intake.

8. When cereals are allowed, these can be taken with fruit juices, sugar, maple syrup, or caramelized sugar.

9. If you are on a cereal-free diet, you should take plenty of tapioca cooked with specified fruits and plenty of sugar, in order to increase weight.

10. If you are underweight or have a tendency to lose weight, large amounts of cooked tapioca should be taken with each meal, and possibly before going to bed or between meals in order to increase your caloric intake.

11. Moreover, plenty of potatoes, sweet and white as allowed, should be eaten. They can be baked, boiled, or fried in specified

oils. You should learn to take them with oil, particularly if weight maintenance is a problem.

12. You can also cook sweet potatoes with maple syrup or sugar, Southern style.

13. The starchy vegetables (as allowed) such as peas, beans, lima beans and squash will help to increase weight if taken in large quantities.

14. If weight decreases in spite of following these directions, be sure to discuss the situation with your physician, or if away from town, be sure to write for further advice.

INSTRUCTIONS FOR THE ESTABLISHMENT OF ENVIRONMENTAL CONTROL*

In order to decrease the possibility of inhaling various dusts, pollens, and other allergens from the air of your homes, it is necessary to prepare your bedroom and sitting room in the following manner.

1. The curtains should be taken down, and either well shaken or freshly laundered. All surfaces of roller shades or blinds should be wiped free from dust.

2. Carpets and underpads should be removed. Floors should be thoroughly cleaned and washable small rugs should be used.

3. The ceiling, walls, picture moulding, window frames, and all woodwork should be wiped down preferably with slightly damp cloths in order to remove all visible and invisible dust thereon.

4. All surfaces of furniture, the springs of the mattress, the frame of the bed, the backs and surfaces of all pictures should be wiped with damp cloths.

5. When moderate dust susceptibility is suspected, the pillows of the beds in the room should be covered with three pillow slips, one being put on one way, another the opposite way, and the third one in the original direction. The mattress should be wrapped in old sheets. The bedding should consist of well washed old woolen blankets or well washed cotton blankets if so ordered by the doctor. No comforters, feather beds, or feather or down comforters should be on the bed.

6. No overstuffed furniture should be left in the room. Day beds or couches, especially, should be taken out of the bedroom, and all plants and flowers should be excluded. Attention should be given to the flowers, vines, and shrubbery which may be close to the house or in gardens within 10 or 15 feet from the windows of the bedroom. In general, such flowers should frequently be

* For further discussion of environmental control, see page 31.

cut, and the vines and shrubbery should be pruned down if indications of possible allergy to them exist. Possible allergy to dusts from flowers, shrubs, animals, birds, or dusts from roofs in adjoining yards must be considered.

7. For patients who are extremely sensitive to house dust and particularly when mattress or feather dust allergy is suspected, covers for mattress and pillows may be ordered. These may be obtained from a manufacturer (see page 32) who makes them according to the measurements of the mattress and pillows, or they may be made by the patient from thin rubberized cloth obtained from department stores. A good quality of such cloth with a rubberized surface on one side can be obtained at approximately 50 cents a yard. Such covers should be made with long flaps on the ends so that they can be turned over several times and pinned, securely. The same long flaps should be made on the pillow slips. A better arrangement is to sew a zipper on the end to prevent the escape of dust.

8. Careful attention should be paid to the dust control of the sitting and living rooms which are used by the patient. The overstuffed furniture and rugs should be vacuumed very carefully. Curtains and drapes should be thoroughly cleaned and walls, woodwork, and floors should be wiped at frequent intervals to eliminate all possible dust. All animals, flowers, and plants should be removed from the house unless specially allowed by the physician.

9. If marked sensitization to house dust or the dust from upholstered furniture or drapes is present, a small room which is devoid of all overstuffed furniture or carpets should be kept for the patient's use while he is reading or working at home.

QUESTIONNAIRE FOR THE ALLERGIC PATIENT[1]

NAME:
ADDRESS:
AGE:
REFERRED BY:

I. ASTHMA:
    1. Do you have asthma?
    2. Describe a typical attack.
    3. Age and date when asthma began.
    4. How often do attacks occur? Usual duration?
    5. What season are symptoms worse?

[1] Adapted from that by Vaughan, W. T.: Practice of Allergy, St. Louis, C. V. Mosby & Co., 1934.

QUESTIONNAIRE FOR THE ALLERGIC PATIENT
(Continued)

I. ASTHMA:

6. If seasonal, give date of occurrence. Are they becoming more frequent, lasting longer?
7. Are you entirely well between attacks?
8. Is there much coughing?
9. Do you raise sputum? What color: whitish, yellowish, or greenish? How much?
10. When did the last or present attack begin?
11. What time of day do symptoms occur? Only at night?
12. Are you better on hot or cold days? Is there any relationship to fog or wind?
13. In what part of the country or city have you been free from trouble? For how long? Does change of residence in the same city give relief? Are you better at the seashore or in the mountains?
14. Have you ever had croup? When? Describe in detail.
15. Do you have bronchitis? Describe attacks, time of occurrence, frequency, etc.
16. Do any of the following cause asthma?
    House dust?
    Road or street dust?
    Any kind of smoke?
    Flowers of any kind?
    Face powders or other cosmetics?
    Any vapors or peculiar odors?
    Contact with animals such as cats, dogs, sheep, cattle, horses, goats, canaries, chickens, ducks or geese?
    Contact with crowds?
    Going to theaters?
    Going into any particular buildings?
    Going into cellars or musty places?
17. Does your trouble come with head colds? If so, is this always true?
18. Are your symptoms related to:
    Menstrual periods?
    Fatigue?
    Emotional upsets?
19. What treatment have you had? Give details.
20. What drugs or remedies do you use for relief? Describe their effects. Are you sensitive to any drugs or medicines? What are they? What symptoms do they produce? How soon after taking?
21. Have you used adrenalin (epinephrine)?
22. Have you ever had skin tests?

II. ENVIRONMENT:

1. How long have you lived in your present neighborhood?
2. What trees are in this locality?
3. Are there open fields?

QUESTIONNAIRE FOR THE ALLERGIC PATIENT

(Continued)

II. ENVIRONMENT:

4. What weeds are in this locality?
5. Any special kind of insects?
6. What factories within a mile?
7. What flowers near the house?
8. What grasses in the lawn?
9. What pets in or around the house?
10. Do they come into the house?
11. Any livestock nearby?
12. How far is the barn from the house?
13. What feeds, hay, grains, etc., are kept in the barn?
14. How old is your house or apartment? Is it damp or sunny? Is the cellar damp? Length of residence in this house?
15. Do you have trouble only at home?
16. How is the house heated?
17. How is it cleaned (vacuum, broom)?
18. Are there mice or rats?
19. What flowers or plants are kept in the house?
20. Do you always sleep in the same bedroom? Do you sleep alone? In a room alone?
21. Of what is your pillow made? Your mattress?
22. What kind of covers do you have? Any down comforts?
23. What kind of floor coverings?
24. Have you many pictures and furniture in the room?
25. How is the room ventilated?

III. HAY FEVER:

1. Do you have symptoms of hay fever?
2. Age and date of onset.
3. Do you have itching of the roof of the mouth? The eyes? The throat? Inside of nose? Deep in the ears? Between shoulder blades? On the skin?
4. Do your eyes water frequently? Are they often irritated?
5. Can you detect odors easily? Can you taste well? Is your nose frequently stopped up?
6. How often do symptoms occur? How long do they last?
7. Are they becoming more frequent and persistent?
8. Are symptoms limited to any yearly season? If so, when?
9. When are they the worst?
10. Is there any change from one season to another? If so, how?
11. Are you worse day or night?
12. Relationship to daily activities?
13. Do you have attacks of uncontrollable sneezing? When?
14. Do you know any cause for your symptoms? See causes related to asthma, Section I, 16.
15. Age and date of onset of symptoms?
16. Are you subject to head colds or sinus trouble? How many each year?
17. Do they differ from hay fever as described?

QUESTIONNAIRE FOR THE ALLERGIC PATIENT
(*Continued*)

III. HAY FEVER:

18. Character of discharge from nose during colds? Amount, color, consistency.
19. How long do they last?
20. What season do they occur?
21. Do you have wheezing, cough or tightness in the chest during colds or hay fever?

IV. SKIN:

1. Have you ever had eczema or any chronic skin eruption? Describe it. Where did it begin and how did it spread?
2. Is it constant or periodic? Of sudden or gradual onset?
3. Is there seasonal variation?
4. Any chronologic association with home or other contacts?
5. What makes it worse? Foods, clothing, menses, illness and remedies, miscellaneous things?
6. What have you done for it—internal and external medicaments and treatments?
7. What medications do you use (proprietary or prescribed) for headaches, constipation, "acid in the system," "blood purifiers," "tonics," for sleeplessness, nervousness, coughs, menstrual periods? Bromo-Seltzer? Bromo Quinine? Iodized salt? Other medication, internal or external, proprietary or prescribed?
8. What cosmetics do you use—scalp tonics, wave-sets, powder, lipstick, rouge, beauty creams, freckle creams, wrinkle removers, perfumes, soaps, bath salts, astringent lotions, depilatories, nail polishes, deodorants, massages, etc.?
9. Any used by others at home?
10. Applied at beauty parlor or elsewhere?
11. What occupational or avocational contacts do you have—at work (principal substances handled, incidental substances such as cleaners, are they liquid or solids)—at home (cleaners, insecticides, professional exterminators, pets, plants, substances used in their care, furniture, drapes, clothing—new, cleaned, dyed—hobbies, photography, stamps, golf, cards, other games), miscellaneous?
12. Have you had urticaria (hives, nettle rash)? When? Recognized cause?
13. Are you bothered by itching of the skin? When? Cause? Relieved by? Parts of skin involved?
14. Have you any other skin eruption? Describe it.
15. Are you susceptible to poison ivy or poison oak?

V. HEADACHES:

1. Are you subject to frequent headaches? Character and duration? Age and date of onset? Frequency of recurrence?
2. What portion of the head is involved?
3. What time of day do they occur? Ever begin at night?

QUESTIONNAIRE FOR THE ALLERGIC PATIENT
(Continued)

V. HEADACHES:
   4. To what have you attributed them?
   5. What gives you relief?
   6. Have you had sick headaches (migraine)? Give frequency of occurrence. Cause if possible. Confined to one side? Which?
   7. Do you begin with eye symptoms, streaks of light, flashes, etc.?
   8. Associated stomach symptoms?
   9. What gives you relief?

VI. GASTRO-INTESTINAL:
   1. Do you have any indigestion? Nausea? Vomiting? Full feeling? Belching? Gas in lower bowels? Cramping or colicky pain in abdomen? Give locations.
   2. Do symptoms occur in attacks? Are they persistent or chronic?
   3. Are you entirely well between attacks?
   4. Are you constipated? Frequency of bowel movements? Character of bowel movements, hard, soft but formed, mushy or watery. Do you use cathartics or enemas?
   5. Do you pass mucus in the stools? How often? Have you been told you had colitis?
   6. Do bowel movements give relief of symptoms?
   7. Have you ever been told you had chronic appendicitis? Have you ever had acute appendicitis? Has your appendix been removed?
   8. Do you suspect any food as cause of symptoms? Name them.
   9. Do you have canker sores? Any itching around rectum? Any relation to above symptoms?

VII. GENITO-URINARY:
   1. Do you have attacks of frequent urination? Bladder pains? So-called kidney colic? Any bladder trouble? Burning on urination? Describe in detail.

VIII. NEUROMUSCULAR:
   1. Do you have low blood-pressure? What is your usual blood-pressure?
   2. Have you ever had convulsions or epileptic seizures? Spells of unconsciousness? Describe.
   3. Do you tire easily? Have you muscle soreness? Attacks of extreme fatigue or sleepiness in the daytime? Do you have nightmares? Are you troubled with sleeplessness? Give details.

IX. DIET:
   1. Do any particular foods cause your trouble?
   2. What symptoms do they produce?
   3. Any particular food dislikes? Reason for dislike? What symptoms do they produce?
   4. For what foods have you a special craving?

QUESTIONNAIRE FOR THE ALLERGIC PATIENT
(Continued)

IX. DIET:

    5. Do particular combinations of foods cause trouble? Does overeating increase symptoms?

    6. Have you been on any special dietary restrictions for your trouble? What were these diets? Did they benefit you? If so, how? Any other benefits or harmful effects?

    7. What is your average diet—average daily helpings of fruits, vegetables, meats. Average daily amount of wheat, milk and egg products. Accessory foods such as cod liver oil?

X. OCCUPATION:

Describe your occupation, giving daily routine and places you visit. Any regular contacts in your daily routine that you might suspect? Is your place of business well ventilated? How heated? Dusty? Flowers or plants in your place of business?

XI. MISCELLANEOUS:

    1. Have you had any roentgen-ray photographs of your chest? By whom? What did it show?

    2. Have you had roentgen-ray photographs of your sinuses? By whom? What did they show?

    3. What other roentgen-ray photographs have you had made? What did they show?

    4. Have you had any operations on your nose and throat? Name each. Give date of operation, reason for it, and results.

    5. What further remarks do you care to make that you think may be of interest or help?

XII. RESIDENCES:

Give residences and approximate time in each since birth.

XIII. PAST HISTORY:

    1. What diseases have you had?

    2. How is your general health?

XIV. FAMILY HISTORY:

List the occurrence of asthma, hay fever, nasal trouble, hives, eczema, headaches, chronic indigestion, and migraine in your parents, grandparents, aunts, uncles, brothers, sisters and children.

THE FOLLOWING HISTORY FORM HAS BEEN USEFUL IN THE FREE CLINIC. IT CAN BE FILLED BY A NURSE OR TRAINED WORKER AND AMPLIFIED BY THE PHYSICIAN

HISTORY OF ALLERGY

Name   S.W.M.   Age   Clinic No.

Present Illness: Asthma, hay fever, repeated head or bronchial colds, hives, angioneurotic edema, eczema, migraine, headaches, gastro-intestinal symptoms, constipation, mucous colitis, pruritis ani (underline positive complaints).

Bronchial Asthma: Age of onset   ; Attacks: frequency   ; duration of wheezing   ; of coughing   . Between attacks: coughing 1, 2, 3, 4; wheezing—constant, with exertion, nocturnal. Perennial occurrence. Exaggeration during spring, summer, fall, winter. Sneezing 1, 2, 3, 4; mucoid, muco-purulent, purulent. Itching of eyes, nose, mouth. During attacks: fever; nausea or vomiting. Environmental influences and effect of dust, animal emanations, pollens, occupational contacts, effect of changes in climate, etc.

General Comments:

Hay Fever: Age of onset   . Since onset: constant, varying, increasing in severity. Perennial   . Occurrence in spring, summer, fall, winter. Sneezing 1, 2, 3, 4. Nasal congestion 1, 2, 3, 4. Discharge: watery, mucoid, purulent. Itching: eyes, nose, throat, ears, skin. Susceptibility to house dust   ; orris root   ; flowers   ; other occupational or environmental dust. Associated with asthma, coughing, dermatitis. Effect of diet or foods on symptoms.

Susceptibility to colds or bronchitis. Frequency and seasonal occurrence.

Hives, Angioneurotic Edema. Age of onset   , duration and distribution.

Eczema. Age of onset   , duration and distribution.

Migraine. Recurrent headaches. Age of onset   , duration   , frequency   . Associated with nausea, vomiting, toxicity, gastro-intestinal symptoms.

Gastro-intestinal Symptoms: Canker sores, coated tongue, sour stomach, distention, nausea or vomiting, cramping, abdominal pain or soreness (up. rt., l. rt., up. left, l. left, epigastr., mid., lower), diarrhea, constipation, mucous colitis, pruritus ani.

History of Colic in Infancy: Digestive disturbances or indigestion in childhood.

Food idiosyncrasies or dislikes: Definite foods productive of symptoms.

Drug idiosyncrasies: Aspirin, quinine, barbitals, ipecac, opiates, etc.

Effect of climatic changes: Note effects. Beneficial locations.

Susceptibility to poison oak or other plants:

Residences:

Family History: Occurrence of asthma, hay fever, hives, angioneurotic edema, migraine, recurrent headaches, repeated colds, coughs or catarrh, chronic indigestion, constipation.

Past Illnesses: Tonsillitis, teeth—out, infected, roentgen-rayed—when?

Operations: Tonsillectomy: Nasal operations (how many):
Antral operations:

HISTORY OF THE ALLERGIC PATIENT

The systematic recording of the history expedites the diagnosis. It may be recorded under the following headings:

1. Bronchial manifestations: Onset, frequency, periodicity, and chronicity of the attacks or persistent symptoms, the amount and character of the sputum, frequency and degree of cough, fever, complications, and former history of bronchial symptoms.

2. Nasal and Sinusal Symptoms: Duration, amount, and degree of seasonal or perennial nasal congestion, blocking, sneezing, itching, nasal or postnasal discharge, sinusal congestion or pain, and former history of head colds or sinusitis.

3. Dermatoses: Onset, duration, and distribution of allergic dermatitis (eczema), contact dermatitis, urticaria, or angioneurotic edema during life, with possible etiologic comment.

4. Gastro-intestinal Symptoms: Occurrence of canker sores and other oral, gastro-intestinal, and abdominal symptoms with their duration, degree, and characteristics, and possible relation to allergy.

5. Recurrent headaches, migraine, biliousness, fatigue, or "toxic states."

6. Genito-urinary, cardio-vascular, glandular, nervous, or psycho-neurotic disturbances, with data for or against allergy as a primary or complicating cause.

7. Dietary History: Dislikes or disagreements for foods of all types, and habits of eating. Questions such as, "Do you drink milk, eat eggs, or spinach?" may suggest allergy, digestive inefficiency, whims or fancies, or psychoneuroses as causes. Potential or active nutritional deficiencies must be recognized as emphasized by Minot.

8. Drug History: Possible allergy to medicaments used even infrequently.

9. Environmental History: The kinds of carpets, curtains, furnishings, mattresses, pillows, bedding, furs, clothings, animals, plants, flowers, cosmetics, toilet accessories, and other similar information concerning the living, sleeping, working, and recreational environments. Likewise, the names of trees, shrubs, flowers, the character of the surrounding region, whether built up or in the country, its proximity to barns, animals, fields, orchards, forests, or marshes, the amount and character of dusts, and similar information.

Family History: Bronchial, nasal, cutaneous, gastro-intestinal, or other symptoms, especially migraine, recurrent headache, toxic or bilious states in several generations and progeny, with a record of possible familial ingestant, inhalation, or contact sensitizations; other usual information concerning familial diseases, longevity, and dietary habits.

Residences: Their possible relation to allergy.

Past History: Past or present infections or illnesses not noted above.

Menstrual History and the possible influence of allergy.

Operations: Year and results of operations, especially on the nose and throat.

Habits: Amount of tobacco and alcohol and their influence on allergy.

Chart for the Graphic Recording of the Manipulation of Elimination Diets

DATE	8/9	1/6
RICE	✓	
CORN	✓	
TAPIOCA	✓	
RYE		
OATS		
WHEAT		
LAMB	✓	
CHICKEN	✓	
BACON	✓	
BEEF		✓
TURKEY		
SALMON		
HALIBUT		

DATE	8/9	1/6
LETTUCE	✓	
SPINACH	✓	
CARROT	✓	
SQUASH	✓	
ASPARAGUS	✓	
PEA	✓	
ARTICHOKE	✓	
TOMATO	✓	✓
BEET	✓	✓
STRING BEAN		✓
CELERY	✓	✓
AVOCADO		
LIMA BEAN		
POTATO (WHITE)		

DATE	8/9	1/6
LEMON	✓	
PEAR	✓	
PEACH	✓	
PINEAPPLE	✓	
APRICOT	✓	
PRUNE	✓	
PLUM		
GRAPEFRUIT		✓
ORANGE		
APPLE		
BANANA		
CANTALOUPE		
WATERMELON		
GRAPE		

DATE	8/9	1/6
SUGAR	✓	
KARO	✓	
MAPLE SYRUP	✓	
MAZOLA OIL	✓	
WESSON OIL		✓
OLIVE OIL	✓	
OLIVE	✓	
SALT	✓	✓
PEPPER		
EGG		
MILK		
BUTTER		
CREAM		

7/1 To eat all types of food. 8/6 To resume diet as ordered on 6/8.

This chart, as described on page 146 allows the graphic recording of the use of the "elimination diets" or other methods of diet trial. When foods are added, a date in the space opposite the food may be used if desired, or a check may be inserted. If a food is removed a zero, together with the date, should be recorded. Foods other than those printed, such as potato, cabbage, dates, various nuts, etc., may be written in the spaces at the end of each column.

GENERAL DIRECTIONS FOR THE ADMINISTRATION OF POLLEN ANTIGENS

For————————————————————————————————————

———————————————————————————————————————19——

My dear Dr.————————————————————————————————

These solutions must be administered at intervals as indicated in the accompanying schedule. THE DOSE MUST BE ACCURATELY MEASURED WITH A TUBERCULIN SYRINGE AND CAREFULLY INJECTED SUBCUTANEOUSLY UNDER STERILE PRECAUTIONS. The injection should be made just under the deep layers of the skin itself in the outerside of the upper arm posterior to its midline, this area being free from superficial large veins. THE SOLUTIONS MUST BE KEPT IN A REFRIGERATOR OR THEY WILL DETERIORATE.

The normal local reaction after a pollen injection consists of a tender reddened area 1 to 3 inches in diameter, occurring within twelve hours after the injection.

With increasing doses, especially during the pollen season, constitutional general reactions may arise, evidenced by mild or severe urticaria, hay fever, coughing or asthma occurring within one to two hours after treatment. The patient should wait in your office for twenty to thirty minutes after each injection and if any sign of a general reaction occurs he should receive an injection of a fresh solution of 1 to 1000 epinephrine or adrenalin, varying from 0.2 to 1 cc. according to the severity of the reaction and the age of the patient. This dose should be repeated every five to thirty minutes until symptoms are relieved. If reactions occur after the patient leaves your office he should take 1 or 2 25-mg. ephedrine capsules (which he should carry with him) and immediately return to your office for adrenalin therapy. A tourniquet applied above the site of injection loosened momentarily every few minutes and kept in place for twenty to thirty minutes will lessen the degree of reaction.

If the patient has had a constitutional reaction, a dose smaller than the one which gave the constitutional reaction must be administered, and the treatment may have to be increased more slowly than is indicated in the schedule. During the pollen season it is often impossible to make much increase in dosage.

During the pollen season, tolerance for the larger doses may be impaired as evidenced by increasing local reactions or the production of symptoms by the injections. Co-seasonal therapy is then indicated with small doses (0.1 cc.) of the 1 to 50, 1 to 500, 1 to 5000 or the 1 to 50,000 dilution given every one to three days. The dose controlling such seasonal symptoms varies with the patient. Daily doses, especially if the weaker solutions are used, may be necessary. As symptoms are controlled and the height of the pollen season is past, the doses may again be increased as rapidly as tolerance permits.

When two or more antigens are sent simultaneously, each one must be measured and administered separately. One antigen should be given in the outer and upper side of one arm, and the other antigen administered in the outer and upper side of the opposite arm, alternating arms from one visit to the next in order to desensitize both arms to each antigen.

If there is any other information which you require in this treatment we shall be glad to have you communicate with us.

Schedule I for Antigen Therapy

(Antigen to be administered subcutaneously every ——————— days with
tuberculin syringe and a 26 gauge ½ inch hypodermic needle.)

1st injection	0.03 cc. (3/100 cc.) of dilution 1–5000			
2d "	0.05 cc. (5/100 cc.)	"	"	
3d "	0.10 cc.	"	"	
4th "	0.20 cc.	"	"	
5th "	0.30 cc.	"	"	
6th "	0.40 cc.	"	"	
7th "	0.05 cc.	"	1–500	
8th "	0.10 cc.	"	"	
9th "	0.20 cc.	"	"	
10th "	0.30 cc.	"	"	
11th "	0.40 cc.	"	"	
12th "	0.05 cc.	"	1–50	
13th "	0.10 cc.	"	"	
14th "	0.15 cc.	"	"	
15th "	0.20 cc.	"	"	
16th "	0.25 cc.	"	"	
17th "	0.30 cc.	"	"	
18th "	0.35 cc.	"	"	
19th "	0.40 cc.	"	"	
20th "	0.45 cc.	"	"	
21st "	0.50 cc.	"	"	
22d "	0.55 cc.	"	"	
23d "	0.60 cc.	"	"	
24th "	0.65 cc.	"	"	
25th "	0.70 cc.	"	"	
26th "	0.75 cc.	"	"	
27th "	0.80 cc.	"	"	

Schedule II for Antigen Therapy

(Antigen to be administered subcutaneously every ——————— days with
a tuberculin syringe and a 26 gauge ½ inch hypodermic needle.)

1st injection	0.05 cc. (5/100 cc.) of dilution 1–5000			
2d "	0.10 cc.	"	"	
3d "	0.15 cc.	"	"	
4th "	0.20 cc.	"	"	
5th "	0.25 cc.	"	"	
6th "	0.30 cc.	"	"	
7th "	0.35 cc.	"	"	
8th "	0.40 cc.	"	"	
9th "	0.45 cc.	"	"	
10th "	0.05 cc.	"	1–500	
11th "	0.10 cc.	"	"	
12th "	0.15 cc.	"	"	
13th "	0.20 cc.	"	"	
14th "	0.25 cc.	"	"	
15th "	0.30 cc.	"	"	
16th "	0.35 cc.	"	"	
17th "	0.40 cc.	"	"	
18th "	0.45 cc.	"	"	

Schedule II for Antigen Therapy—*(Continued)*

19th injection 0.05 cc. (5/100 cc.) of dilution 1–50
20th	"	0.075 cc.	" "
21st	"	0.10 cc.	" "
22d	"	0.125 cc.	" "
23d	"	0.15 cc.	" "
24th	"	0.175 cc.	" "
25th	"	0.20 cc.	" "
26th	"	0.225 cc.	" "
27th	"	0.25 cc.	" "
28th	"	0.275 cc.	" "
29th	"	0.30 cc.	" "
30th	"	0.325 cc.	" "
31st	"	0.35 cc.	" "
32d	"	0.375 cc.	" "
33d	"	0.40 cc.	" "
34th	"	0.425 cc.	" "
35th	"	0.45 cc.	" "
36th	"	0.475 cc.	" "
37th	"	0.50 cc.	" "
38th	"	0.525 cc.	" "
39th	"	0.55 cc.	" "
40th	"	0.575 cc.	" "
41st	"	0.60 cc.	" "

Continue with this last dose at weekly intervals until all the 1–50 dilution is exhausted.

If a local reaction larger than 3 inches in diameter occurs within twenty-four hours, the dose should be repeated at the next treatment. If a constitutional reaction occurs, the dose should be reduced to the previous one or smaller if the reaction is very severe. If no local reaction occurs, the treatment can be carried out faster than indicated, by skipping alternate doses, providing the injections do not activate or exaggerate symptoms. Modification of treatment during the pollen season is discussed in the general directions.

Supplemental Schedule for More Dilute Solutions
Schedule for Antigen Therapy

(Antigen to be administered subcutaneously every ———— days with a tuberculin syringe and a 26 gauge ½ inch hypodermic needle.)

1st injection 0.10 cc. (1/10 cc.) of dilution 1–5,000,000
2d	"	0.20 cc.	" "
3d	"	0.30 cc.	" "
4th	"	0.40 cc.	" "
5th	"	0.50 cc.	" "
6th	"	0.10 cc.	" 1–500,000
7th	"	0.20 cc.	" "
8th	"	0.30 cc.	" "
9th	"	0.40 cc.	" "
10th	"	0.50 cc.	" "
11th	"	0.10 cc.	" 1–50,000
12th	"	0.20 cc.	" "
13th	"	0.30 cc.	" "
14th	"	0.40 cc.	" "
15th	"	0.50 cc.	" "

FOOD DIARY

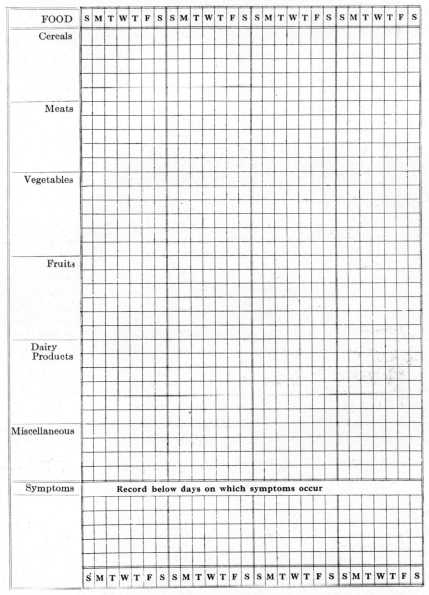

Foods can be listed on the left hand side of the chart and checks made on days they are taken. The symptoms can be listed under "symptoms" and the days they occur can be indicated by checks.

Food Protein Groups* (Vaughan)

1. Walnut
   Pecan
2. Swiss chard
   Beet
   Spinach
   Radish
   Turnip
   Cabbage
   Cauliflower
   Mustard
4. Blackberry
   Strawberry
   Raspberry
5. Almond
   Cherry
   Apricot
   Plum
   Peach
6. Pea
   Lima bean

Kidney bean
Lentil
Peanut
String bean
7. Lemon
   Orange
   Grapefruit
8. Grape
   Okra
9. Cocoa
10. Parsley
    Celery
    Parsnip
    Carrot
11. Sweet potato
12. Tomato
    Potato, Irish
    Eggplant
13. Pumpkin
    Squash

Cantaloupe
Cucumber
Watermelon
14. Lettuce
    Artichoke
15. Rye
16. Wheat
17. Barley
18. Oat
19. Rice
20. Corn
21. Onion
    Garlic
    Asparagus
22. Banana
    Ginger
23. Apple
    Pear

* Test solutions 23 to 28 represent animal foods.

Botanical Classification of Edible Plants (Vaughan)

Family.	Genus.	Species.	Common name.
Monocotyledones.			
Graminæ	Triticum	sativum	Wheat
	Secale	cereale	Rye
	Hordeum	vulgare	Barley
	Avena	sativa	Oat
	Oryza	sativa	Rice
	Zea	mays	Corn
Palmaceæ	Cocos	nucifera	Cocoanut
	Phoenix	dactylifera	Date
Bromeliaceæ	Ananus	sativus	Pineapple
Liliaceæ	Allium	cepa	Onion
		sativum	English garlic
	Asparagus	officinalis	Asparagus
Musaceæ	Musa	sapientum	Banana
Zinziberaceæ	Zinziber	officinale	Ginger
Dicotyledones			
Moraceæ	Morus	nigra	Black mulberry
	Ficus	carica	Fig
Polygonaceæ	Fagopyrum	vulgare	Buckwheat
	Pheum	rhaponticum	Rhubarb
Juglandaceæ	Juglans	nigra	Black walnut
		regia	English walnut
	Carya	olivæformis	Pecan
		alba	Hickory
Betulaceæ	Corylus	avellana	Hazelnut, filbert
	Castanea	dentata	Chestnut
Chenopodiaceæ	Spinacia	oleracea	Spinach
	Beta	vulgaris	Beet
		cycla	Swiss chard
Grossulariaceæ	Ribes	vulgare	Currant
		ocyacanthoides	Gooseberry
Cruciferæ	Raphanus	sativus	Radish
	Radicula	armoracia	Horseradish
		nasturtium aquatium	Water cress
	Brassica	rapa	Turnip
		campestris	Rutabaga
		alba	White mustard
		nigra	Brown mustard
		oleracea capitata	Cabbage
		oleracea acephala	Kale

Botanical Classification of Edible Plants (Vaughan)—*Continued.*

Family.	Genus.	Species.	Common name.
		Dicotyledones	
Cruciferæ	Brassica	oleracea gemmifera	Brussels sprout
		oleracea caulo-rapa	Kohlrabi
		oleracea botrytis	Cauliflower
			(Broccoli)
Rosaceæ	Rubus	nigrobaccus	Blackberry
		occidentalis	Black raspberry
		strigosus	Red raspberry
	Fragaria	chiloensis	Strawberry
Pomaceæ	Malus	sylvestris	Apple
	Pyrus	communis	Pear
Drupaceæ	Prunus	amygdalus	Almond
		domestica	Plum, prune
		avium	Cherry
		armeniaca	Apricot
		persica	Peach
Leguminosæ	Pisum	sativum	Pea
	Phaseolus	vulgaris	Kidney bean
		lunatus	Lima bean
	Lens	esculenta	Lentil
	Acharis	hypogæa	Peanut
Rutaceæ	Citrus	limonia	Lemon
		grandis	Grapefruit
		sinensis	Common orange
Anacardiaceæ	Pistacia	vera	Pistachio nut
Vitaceæ	Vitis	vinifera	Grape, raisin
Malvaceæ	Gossypium	hirsutum	Cotton seed
		barbadense	
	Hibiscus	esculentus	Okra, gumbo
Sterculiaceæ	Theobroma	cacao	Cocoa
Theaceæ	Thea	sinensis	Tea
Umbelliferæ	Daucus	carota	Carrot
	Pastinaca	sativa	Parsnip
	Apium	petroselinum	Parsley
		graveolens	Celery
Vacciniaceæ	Gaylussacia	resinosa	Huckleberry
	Vaccinium	macrocarpon	Cranberry
Oleaceæ	Olea	europœa	Olive
Convolvulaceæ	Ipomœa	batatas	Sweet potato
Solanaceæ	Solanum	tuberosum	Potato
		melongena	Eggplant
	Lycopersicum	esculentum	Tomato
Rubiaceæ	Coffea	arabica	Coffee

Botanical Classification of Edible Plants (Vaughan)—*Continued.*

Family.	Genus.	Species.	Common name.
		Dicotyledones	
Cucurbitaceæ	Cucurbita	pepo	Pumpkin
		moschata	Winter squash
		maxima	Hubbard squash
	Cucumis	melo	Cantaloupe
		sativus	Cucumber
	Citrullus	vulgaris	Watermelon
Compositæ	Lactuca	sativa	Lettuce
(Chichoriaceæ)			
	Tragopogon	porrifolius	Salsify,
			oyster plant
	Chicorium	intybus	Chicory
		endiva	Endive
Compositæ	Helianthus	tuberosus	Jerusalem
(Asteraceæ)			artichoke
	Cynara	scolymus	Artichoke

Ellis* (1931) published the following supplement to Vaughan's genetic classification of food allergens:

PLANTS.

Common name.	Family.	Genus.	Species.
	Monocotyledones.		
Sorghum	Graminæ	Holcus	sorghum
Leek	Liliaceæ	Allium	parrum
Chive	"	"	schoenoprosum
	Dicotyledones.		
Hops	Moraceæ	Humulus	lupulus
Hazelnut	Betulaceæ	Corylus	americana
Blueberry	Ericaceæ	Vaccinium	corymbosum
Dewberry	Rosaceæ	Rubus	flagellaris
Tangerine	Rutaceæ	Citrus	nobilis
Maple sugar	Aceraceæ	Acer	saccharum
Green and red pepper	Solonaceæ	Capsicum	frutescens
Ground cherry	"	Physalis	pubescens
Yam	Dioscoreaceæ	Dioscorea	batatas
Dill	Umbelliferæ	Anethum	graveolens

EDIBLE ANIMALS.

Invertebrata.
Phyllum Mullusca.

Common name.	Class.	Family.	Genus.	Species.
Abalone (red)	Gastropoda	Haliotidæ	Haliotis	rufescens
Abalone (green)	"	"	"	fulgens
Snail (edible)	"	Helicidæ	Helix	pomatia
Mussel, salt water	Pelecypoda	Mytilidæ	Mytilus	edulis
Mussel, fresh	"	Unionidæ	Unio	(several sp.)
Mussel, fresh	"	"	Anodonta	(several sp.)
Oysters	"	Ostreidæ	Ostrea	virginica
Oysters	"	"	"	lurida
Scallops (common)	"	Pectinidæ	Pecten	irradians
Scallops	"	"	"	islandicus
Scallops (giant)	"	"	"	magellanicus
Clams (soft shell)	"	Myidæ	Mya	arenaria
Clams, razor	"	Solenidæ	Eusis	viredis
Clams, round	"	Veneridæ	Venus	mercenaria
Squid	Cephalopoda	Loliginidæ	Loligo	pealei

Phylum Arthropoda.
Class—Crustacea.

Common name.	Family.	Genus.	Species.
Lobster	Nephropidæ	Homarus	americanus
Lobster (European)	"	"	homarus
Lobster (Norwegian)	"	Nephrops	norwegini
Lobster (Spanish)		Scyllarides	sculptus
Crayfish	Astacidæ	Astacus	nigrescens
Crayfish	"	Cambarus	limosus
Shrimp	Crangonidæ	Crangon	vulgaris
Shrimp, California	"	"	franciscorum
Prawn	Palaemonidæ	Palaemon	vulgaris
Prawn	"	"	serratis
Sou. shrimp and prawn	Peneidæ	Peneus	setiferus
Spiny lobster (Florida crayfish)	Palinuridæ	Palinurus	argus
Crabs, rock	Cancridæ	Cancer	irroratus
Crabs, Jonah	"	"	borealis
Crabs, California	"	"	magister
Crabs, blue	Portunidæ	Callinectes	sapidus
Crabs, lady	"	Ovalipes	ocellatus

* ELLIS, R. V.: Rational Grouping of Food Allergens, Jour. Allergy, **2**, 246, 1931.

(Continued)

Vertebrata.
Class—Pisces.

Common name.	Synonym.	Family.	Genus.	Species.
Anchovy, western		Engraulidæ	Anchovia	delicatissima
Anchovy, California		"	Engraulis	mordax
Bass, black, small mouth		Centrarchidæ	Micropterus	dolomieu
Bass, black, large mouth		"	"	salmoides
Crappie		"	Pomoxis	annularis
Calico bass	Strawberry bass	"	"	sparoides
Rock bass	Goggle eye	"	Ambloplities	rupestris
Bluegill	Blue sunfish	"	Lepomis	pallidus
Butterfish	Harvestfish	Stromateidæ	Pronotus	triacanthus
Harvestfish	Whiting	"	Peprilus	paru
Buffalo, common		Catostomidæ	Ictiobus	cyprinella
Buffalo, white		"	"	bubolus
Drum	Lake carp	"	Carpoides	thompsoni
Sucker, common	White sucker	"	Catostomas	commersoni
Catfish, blue	Mississippi cat	Siluridæ	Ictalurus	furcatus
Channel cat	Spotted cat	Siluridæ	Ictalurus	punctatus
Codfish		Gadidæ	Gadus	callarias
Haddock		"	Melanogrammus	aeglefinus
Flounder (Atlantic)		Pleuonectidæ	Glyptocephalus	cyanoglussus
Flounder (Atlantic)		"	Pleuronectes	americanus
Flounder (Pacific)		"	Platichthys	stellatus
Halibut (Atlantic or Pacific)		"	Hippoglossus	hippoglossus
Halibut (Pacific)		"	Paralichthys	californicus
Pike, wall eyed	Jack salmon	Percidæ	Stizostedion	vitreum
Pike, sand	Sauger	"	"	canadense
Perch, yellow	Ringed perch	"	Perca	flavescens
Pickerel	Common pike	Esoscidæ	Esox	lucius
Muskellunge		"	"	masquinongy
Herring, common		Clupeidæ	Clupeus	larengus
Herring	California herring	"	"	pallasii
Shad, common		"	Alosa	sapidissima
Sardines	Spanish sardine	"	Clupandon	pseudohispanicus
Sardines	California sardine	"	"	ceruleus
Smelts, American		Argentidinidæ	Osmerus	mordaxchthys
Smelts, California		"	"	thaleichthys
Sturgeon, common		Acipenseridæ	Acipenser	sturio
Salmon, pink		Salmonidæ	Oncorhynchus	gorbuscha

Vertebrata.
Class—Pisces.

Common name.	Synonym.	Family.	Genus.	Species.
Salmon, red	Sockeye salmon	Salmonidæ	Oncorhynchus	nerca
Salmon, red	Chinook salmon	"	"	tsacawytscha
Whitefish	Common whitefish	"	Coregonus	clupeiformis
Lake herring	Cisco	"	Argyrosomonas	artedi
Bloater	Silver whitefish	"	"	prognathus
Trout	Rainbow trout	"	Salmo	irideus
Trout	Speckled trout	"	Salvelinus	fontinalis
Lake trout	Mackinaw trout	"	Cristovomer	namaycush
Lake trout	Siscowet	"	"	siscowet
Weakfish	Sea trout	Scienidæ	Cynoscion	regalis
Mackerel	Common mackerel	Scombridæ	Scombrus	scombrus
Mackerel	Chub mackerel	"	"	japonicus
Tuna fish		"	Thunnus	thynnus
Mackerel	Spanish mackerel	"	Scomberomoras	maculatus

Class—Amphibia.

Frog	Bull frog	Ranidæ	Rana	catesbiana

Class—Reptilia.

Turtle	Troosts turtle	Testudinidæ	Chrysempys	troosti
Turtle	Diamond back terrapin	"	Malacoclemnys	palustris

15

(Continued)

Class—Aves.

Chicken	Gallinæ	Gallus	domesticus
Turkey	"	Meleagris	gallopavo—bronze
Turkey	"	"	americana—black
Goose	Anserinæ	Anser	anser
Duck		Anas	domestica
Guinea		Nemida	meleagris
Squab	Columbæ	Columba	livia
Quail	Perdicidæ	Ortyx	virginiana
Quail, mountain	"	Oreortyx	pictus
Quail, California	"	Laphortyx	californicus
Grouse	Tetraonidæ	Tetræ	cupido—prairie chicken
Partridge	"	Bonasa	nubellus

Class—Mammalia.

Common name.	Order.	Family.	Genus.	Species.
Beef	Ungulata	Bovidæ	Bos	taurus
Beef (buffalo)	"	"	"	bison—buffalo
Beef	"	"	"	indicus—Indian cattle
Mutton	"	"	Ovis	aries
Goat	"	"	Capra	?
Reindeer, caribou	"	Cervidæ	Cervus	tarandus
Rabbit	Rodentia	Leporidæ	Lepus	sylvaticus—U. S. cottontail
Rabbit	"	"	"	americanus—American hare
Squirrel	"	Sciuridæ	Sciuris	hudsonicus—red squirrel
Squirrel	"		"	carolinensis—gray squirrel
Squirrel	"		"	niger—fox squirrel

COMPARISON OF UNIT VALUES OF POLLEN EXTRACTS
(According to Tuft)*

Comparable Values of Pollen Extracts

By weight of pollen (Noon unit in 0.001 mg. pollen)	By total nitrogen (Kjeldahl)	By protein nitrogen (Cooke & Stull) units
1 cc. of 1:1,000,000 (1 Noon unit) . .	0.000016	0.64
1 cc. of 1:100,000 (10 units)	0.00016	0.4
1 cc. of 1:10,000 (100 units)	0.0016	64
1 cc. of 1:1000 (1000 units)	0.016	640
1 cc. of 1:100 (10,000 units)	0.16	6400

SERUM ADMINISTRATION AND REACTIONS

Before injecting serum, every patient should be tested for possible serum allergy. Special care is necessary in patients with an allergic history, especially of asthma or nasal allergy, and particularly of nasal or bronchial symptoms arising in proximity to horses, mules, or even to other animals.† An occasional patient

* Tuft, L.: Clinical Allergy, W. B. Saunders Company, Philadelphia, 1937.
† Patients known to be allergic to animal emanations and sera should be immunized to diphtheria and tetanus with alum precipitate toxoids to prevent future emergency serum therapy. (See Active Immunization Against Tetanus, Jour. Am. Med. Assn., **111**, 159, 1938.)

who apparently inherits "natural" horse dander or serum allergy may rapidly develop severe asthma, anaphylactic shock, and may even die with the injection of 1/1000 cc. of serum. Since allergy frequently develops after serum therapy, the number and amount of previous injections of serum must be determined. Acquired sensitization from previous serum therapy or toxin-antitoxin immunization usually produces less serious reactions than arise in animal dander-sensitive patients. Opii and Kahn have shown that the tissues of a patient who has received serum anchor the injected antitoxin so that adequate distant tissue protection is impossible. Larger immunizing doses are necessary in such patients.

Before serum therapy, a scratch or needle puncture test with undiluted serum should be done. If negative in twenty minutes, a drop of serum diluted 1 to 10 with saline solution should be dropped into the eye and an intradermal injection of 0.02 cc. of serum diluted to 1 to 100 with sterile saline should be made. If both these tests are negative, 0.10 cc. of undiluted serum can be given subcutaneously, and in twenty minutes, if no local or general reaction is evident, the immunizing dose can be injected or intravenous serum can be started, giving it slowly, and watching carefully for any evidences of allergic reaction not indicated by history or previous testing.

If an immediate scratch reaction occurs, especially with a history of inhalant allergy to horse dander, serum therapy at times, even when given with the following precautions, is impossible because of the severity of the reaction. In such patients anti-serum from cattle or rabbits may be available. Preliminary tests as outlined in this article and similar care in the injection of such serum, however, are as necessary as they are with horse serum. When such sera are not available and when the danger of tetanus, diphtheria, or other diseases is great, the horse serum administration may be attempted as follows: Scratch or puncture tests should be made with serum dilutions of 1 to 1000, 1 to 10,000, 1 to 100,000 and 1 to 1,000,000. In thirty minutes 0.10 cc. of the dilution which gives no reaction whatsoever can be given intradermally. In extremely sensitive patients a 1 to 1,000,000 or even 1 to 10,000,000 solution might be necessary. In thirty minutes if no local reaction larger than $\frac{1}{2}$ inch in diameter and no evidence of respiratory or cutaneous allergy develop, 0.10 cc. of the same dilution can be given subcutaneously. Every twenty minutes thereafter the dose can be increased as suggested below. Doses may be skipped if increasing evidence of tolerance or desensitization to the serum arises. The initial dose depends on the skin reaction as noted above. All injections should be given in an extremity so that a tourniquet can be applied above the injected area if a rapid allergic reaction arises.

Dilution of serum	Amount injected, cc.	Dilution of serum	Amount injected, cc.
1:100,000,000	0.10	1:100	0.10
"	0.20	"	0.20
"	0.40	"	0.40
1:10,000,000	0.10	"	0.60
"	0.20	1:10	0.10
"	0.40	"	0.20
1:1,000,000	0.10	"	0.40
"	0.20	"	0.60
"	0.40	Undiluted	0.05
1:100,000	0.10	"	0.10
"	0.20	"	0.15
"	0.40	"	0.20
1:10,000	0.10	"	0.30
"	0.20	"	0.40
"	0.40	"	0.60
"	0.60	"	0.80
1:1,000	0.10	"	1.00
"	0.20	"	1.50
"	0.40	"	2.00
"	0.60	"	etc.

As already stated, this schedule may be faster or slower according to the patient's local and general response. Such slow administration is tedious; but if it allows the life saving administration of the serum in the extremely sensitive or naturally allergic patient, it is justified. If the entire schedule as suggested is necessary, twenty-four hours or longer might be required. As stated before, a rare patient cannot be given even the very dilute serum without unjustified danger. Park reported 1 death in every 70,000 injections of serum.

If the scratch reaction is negative and the ocular or the first intradermal test is positive, the injections can be given according to the above schedule starting with the dilution which fails to react by the intradermal test. According to the degree of resultant allergy, the speed of increase must be slower or faster than the printed schedule.

Therapy of immediate reactions: Epinephrine or adrenalin, 1 to 1000, must be immediately available during all serum therapy. Doses of from 0.20 to 1.00 cc. according to age and degree of reaction, may be given subcutaneously every ten to sixty minutes and every one to six hours thereafter until such clinical reactivity subsides. Histaminase, 10 to 30 units three to four times a day may be given by mouth with possible relief to the serum allergy.

Therapy of delayed serum reactions: Erythema, urticaria, angioneurotic edema, pruritus, joint pain, gastro-intestinal symptoms, fever, and the other recognized results of serum disease may occur in a few hours to eight to ten days after the injection. Histaminase in doses noted above may gradually produce relief. Epinephrine or adrenalin subcutaneously in doses as suggested above may also be necessary for one to eight days. At times 1 to 100 epinephrine by inhalation or ephedrine by mouth may be sufficient. For pruritus, colloidal-soda baths, carbolized calamine lotion, or other soothing lotions may be helpful.

Additional serum therapy may be administered providing the interval does not exceed five days. A longer time between injections at times may be productive of allergy. Patients who evidence allergic manifestations after previous serum injections should be reinjected by the same technic as already detailed, special care being taken with patients who show definite allergic reactivity.

USUAL INGREDIENTS IN VARIOUS COMMERCIAL FOODS AND THEIR PRODUCTS

Patients on Elimination or other trial diets must eat no commercial or prepared mixtures of foods unless all ingredients have been actually added to their diets by their physicians. The ingredients in the foods listed below have been obtained from textbooks by Tuft* and Vaughan† and from original sources. Contents of such products may vary from year to year. The government requirement that the ingredients of food products must be printed on wrappers or labels is helpful to patients but their absolute accuracy and the various ingredients listed below must be questioned in many instances.

Baby Foods

The commercial companies, Clapp, Gerber, Heinz, Libby, and Stokeley offer a wide choice of strained and chopped vegetables, puréed fruits, cereal products, soups, and puddings for infants and young children. Vegetables contain only added salt, but the ingredients of other products are printed on the labels.

Borden's Malted Milk—barley malt, wheat flour, whole milk; *Carnrick's Soluble Food*—malted wheat, dried milk, milk sugar; *Diatased Farina*—malted cereal food; *Dryco*—irradiated dried milk; *Dryco (Special)*—rice "polish," vitamin B, irradiated milk; *Farina*—wheat; *Goat's milk*—canned and evaporated by Meyenberg Co., California; *Horlick's Malted Milk*—barley, wheat flour, dried whole milk, malt, $NaHCO_3$; *Karo Syrup*—corn syrup; *Kreme O'Soy*—soy beans, soy oil, calcium phosphate, dextrose;

* Tuft, L.: Clinical Allergy, W. B. Saunders Company, Philadelphia, 1937.
† Vaughan, W. T.: Practice of Allergy, Mosby & Co., St. Louis, 1939.

Mellin's Food—wheat flour, wheat bran, malted barley, potassium bicarbonate; *Moore's Food*—wheat malt; *Mull-Soy*—a milk substitute containing soy bean, soy bean oil, dextrose, sucrose, and minerals (Mueller Laboratories, Baltimore, Md.); *Nestle's Food*—malted whole wheat, malt, dry milk, wheat flour, cod-liver oil; *Pablum*—wheat meal, oatmeal, corn meal, yeast, beef bone, iron, and salt; *Similac*—cow's milk, olive oil, cocoanut oil, cod-liver oil, olive oil lactose; *Stokely's Strained Baby Cereal*—cereal grains, milk, soy bean, salt, yeast; *Sobee*—soy bean, olive oil, arrowroot starch, dextri-maltose, dicalcium phosphate.

BEVERAGES
(*Non-alcoholic*)

Soft drinks contain cane, beet, or corn sugars, colored with artificial or natural colors and flavored with fruit juices or with natural, synthetic, essential oils, usually in carbonated water.

Coca-Cola—caffeine, caramel, essential oils (cinnamon, coriander, lemon, neroli, nutmeg, sweet orange), glycerin, lime juice, phosphoric acid, soluble extracts of coca leaves or kola nuts and water (carbonated); *Cocamalt*—dried skimmed milk, cocoa, barley malt, sucrose, flavoring, dextrose, added Ca, P, Fe, and vitamins A, B$_1$ and D; *Coffee*—often adulterated with chicory and rarely with other roasted nuts or grains. (See page 94.) *Ginger Ale*—carbonated water containing ginger (or ginger extract) and lemon juice (or lemon oil and citric acid), capsicum extract is frequently substituted in part for ginger; *Ovaltine*—barley malt, dried egg and milk cocoa, salt, flavoring, supplemental Ca, P, Fe, vitamins A, B$_1$ and C; *Root Beer*—an extract containing a fermented infusion of root bark and herbs containing essential oils such as sarsaparilla, birch, spruce, wild cherry, spikenard, wintergreen, anise, cassia cloves, lemon, coumarin, vanilla, ginger, with sugar and yeast added and may contain egg to increase foaming; *Sarsaparilla*—caramel, cologne spirits, oils of anise, orange, sassafras, wintergreen, powdered pumice stone, sugar and water.

BEVERAGES
(*Alcoholic*)

Beer (Ale, Stout, Porter)—fermented malted grain, usually barley, though wheat, rye, oats, rice, and corn may be used. Hops (dried flower of the hop vine) are usually added; *Brandy*—distilled from fermented juices of grapes or from peaches, cherries, apricots, apples, and other fruits; *Gin*—distilled from a mixture of wheat, barley, malt, rye and corn. The following flavors may be used: angelica root or seed, aniseed, calamus, caraway, cardamom, cassia (cinnamon), coriander, fennel, juniper berries, lemon peel, licorice root, nutmeg, orange peel, sweet orange, neroli (extract of orange blossom), orris root, sloe berries, turpentine in any combination; *Liqueurs*—sweet liquors made by distilling and mixing various alcohols with essential oils, flavors, and syrups; *Rum*—distilled from cane sugar products; *Whiskey*—distilled from malt, corn, rye, and other cereals. "*Sake*"—Japanese beer made from rice; *Wines*—fermented fruit juices, usually grapes. (See page 90.)

BREAD

Glazing of crusts done with egg and at times with milk. Buckwheat flour is used on the bottom of some breads to prevent burning. The kind of oil, shortening or grease used on the pan and in the bread must be determined from each baker or cook.

Buckwheat Bread—buckwheat, wheat, yeast, and salt and other flours. Milk and egg at times are added; *French Bread*—Cassou's Sour French—salt, water, yeast, malt, and flour; Cassou's Sweet French—salt, water, milk, yeast, malt, and flour; *Hausbrot* or *Tafelbrot*—wheat and rye; *Knupfel* —rye and wheat; *Kommisbrot*—rye (rye flour may have some added wheat); *Lima Bean Bread*—commercial product contains lima bean flour, wheat flour, milk, egg, salt, yeast, in varying proportions. (See page 238 for recipe for bread to be used with elimination diets.) *Oatbread*—oatmeal, wheat flour, potatoes, yeast, salt; *Pumpernickel*—coarse rye flour (20 per cent) bleached, clear rye flour (80 per cent), malt, salt, caramel coloring (like molasses or chicory). Much so-called pumpernickel contains wheat flour; *Rice Bread*—wheat, rice, potato, and often milk; *Rye Bread*—rye, wheat, yeast, and often milk. (See page 248.) *Roman Meal Bread*— ground flaxseed, wheat, milk, and salt; *RyKrisp* (Ralston Company)— Whole rye, salt water; *Soy Bean Bread*—commercial product contains soy bean flour, wheat flour, gluten (wheat) flour, milk, egg, salt, yeast in varying amounts. (For use with elimination diet, see recipes on page 238.) *"Hollywood Bread"*—wheat flour, malt, yeast, salt, honey, caramel, whole rye, oatmeal, soya, gluten, and barley flours, sesame seed, dehydrated vegetables—celery, lettuce, pumpkin, cabbage, carrot, spinach, parsley, sea kelp. *Cassou's Vita-Meal Bread*—wheat, rye, honey, yeast, shortening, oatmeal, sugar, salt, flaxseed, skim milk, malt; *White breads*—wheat flour, sugar, shortening (of various kinds), milk, yeast, salt, molasses may be used; *Bill Baker's Soy Bean Bread*—wheat flour, soy bean flour, skimmed milk, vegetable shortening, honey, salt, yeast; *Potato Bread*—wheat flour, potato flour, milk, shortening, salt, yeast, sugar.

CANDY AND CONFECTIONERY PRODUCTS

The inclusion of chocolate, egg albumen, milk, and butter in varying amounts in most of these products must be remembered. The salesgirl in candy shops rarely knows the ingredients of her merchandise. Only the candy maker, himself, has this information. By law, it should be printed on all candy containers. In addition, cane or beet sugar, corn syrup, honey, molasses, cocoanut oil, palmnut oil, yeast, salt, agar-agar, gum arabic (acacia), gum Tragacanth, Karaya gum, glycerin, artificial color, cocoanut, nuts of various kinds, fruits, raisins, soy albumen, cream of tartar, various flavors and essential oils, are utilized in varying combinations by different manufacturers.

The use of such candies, of course, is forbidden when patients are on elimination diets until the physician includes every ingredient in a given commercial product in the patient's diet. Candy can be made containing various ingredients in the elimination diet. (See recipes on page 244 and 257.)

CANNED FISH

Much fish is packed in various vegetable oils. Spices, at times, are added. It is important to know the exact nature of such oils, spices, etc., before they are eaten by any allergic patient.

CANNED FRUITS

Most canned fruits contain the separate fruit with or without granulated (cane or beet) sugar. *Corn* glucose is occasionally used. The Del Monte products, for instance, are all canned with cane or beet sugar except for figs, to which a little corn syrup is added. The contents must be determined from the label or the company.

CANNED VEGETABLES

Vegetables are canned in water with salt added for seasoning. Artichokes contain citric acid.

CEREALS

Naturally occurring cereal products and flours are discussed on pages 62 to 65. *Beemax*—rye, barley and wheat germ; *Berger's Food*—wheat flour and pancreatic extract; *Brittle Bits*—malted wheat and barley; *California Wheatine*—wheat; *Ceraline Flakes*—corn; *Corn Flakes*—corn, malt extract, sugar and salt; *Cream of Wheat*—Farina with added wheat embryo, Ca, P and Fe; *Cream of Rice*—rice and powdered milk; *Dina-Mite*—oats, bran, flax; *Falona*—wheat, oats, barley, and bean flour; *Force*—malted wheat and barley; *F. S. Granulated Hominy*—corn; *Farina*—wheat; *Grape Nuts and Flakes*—whole wheat flour, malted barley flour, yeast, salt; *Grape Nuts Wheat Meal*—whole wheat, thiamin, sugar, salt, flavoring; *Hecker's Hominy*—corn; *H.O. Co. Hominy*—corn; *Kix* (*Gold Medal*)—cornmeal, tapioca, wheat germ, sugar, salt, vegetable oil, phosphates, iron, vitamins B_1 and G_1; *John Bull Foods*—dried milk and cereals; *Macaroni*—wheat and milk (rice macaroni made by Chinese); *Maltine*—malted barley, wheat, oats, vitamins B and C; *Malt-O-Meal*—farina, toasted malt barley; *Mazuma*—corn; *Muffets*—whole wheat; *Nichol's Snow Whites*—corn; *New Pettijohn's*—whole wheat; *Nutro*—cereal and peanut flour; *Pillsbury's Vites*—wheat; *Popcorn*—butter or salad oil such as cottonseed may be used; *Postum Cereal*—whole wheat, bran, cane sugar, molasses; *Post's Bran*—Bran flakes and other parts of wheat flour, malt syrup and salt; *Post-O-Wheat*—wheat, sugar, salt, flavoring; *Quaker's Crackels*—corn, wheat, oats; *Quaker's Farina*—wheat; *Quaker's Oats*—oats; *Quaker's Crackles*—wheat, oats, brown sugar, salt; *Ralston's Health Breakfast Food*—wheat. *Rice Biscuits*—(Battle Creek Food Co.)—rice, yeast, sugar, salt; *Roman Meal*—ground flaxseed, rye, wheat, bran, salt; *Savoy and Moore's Food*—wheat flour and malt; *Sperry Wheat Hearts*—farina with wheat germ added; *Spaghetti*—wheat and milk; *Steinhardt's Infortina*—diastased cereals, dried milk, lactose cane sugar; *Swan's Potato Starch Flour*—potato; *U. S. Health Food*—ground flaxseed.

PREPARED FLOUR

The ingredients of such flours for pancakes, waffles, biscuits, and so-called self-rising flours are listed on all packages by law. The listing of the many kinds, therefore, is superfluous. It must be remembered that powdered milk or buttermilk and shortening of various types are often included. *Swansdown Cake Flour* contains endosperm of wheat.

CHEESES

(See discussion of cheeses on page 70)

American Brie, Camembert, Cheshire, Cheshire Stilton, Edam, Emmenthaler, Gorgonzola, Gammalost, Gruyère, Limburger, Neufchatel, Parmesan, Pineapple, and Stilton—all from cow's milk; Sagecheese is American cheese flavored; *Ged Ost*—goat's milk; *Gorgonzola*—cow's or goat's milk; *Kraft*—processed cheese; *Lattinini*—tame buffalo's milk; *Lipton*—goat's milk seasoned with pepper and spices; *Mantasia*—cow's or goat's milk; *Roquefort*—sheep's milk.

FERMENTED MILK PRODUCTS

Koumiss—fermented milk of mares or asses; also cow's milk fermented by yeast; *Kefir*—fermented cow's or goat's milk; *Leben*—cow's milk fermented by special coagulant.

COOKIES AND CRACKERS
(*Commercial*)

Many varieties are manufactured containing varying amounts of wheat, corn, milk, butter, egg, chocolate, lard, vegetable oils, soda, salt, yeast, flavors, coloring, molasses, sugar, corn syrup, and other ingredients. The pure food law now requires all ingredients printed on labels, and the manufacturer will always send such information on request. Products are made by various companies free of egg, milk, or wheat. Other ingredients must be known and must only be included in the patient's diet by the physician's order.

DESSERTS

Blanc Mange—Irish moss, milk, flavoring. *Cornstarch*—ground rice and arrowroot are often used; *Custard*—eggs, milk, sugar, flavoring; *D-Zerta*—gelatin, citric acid, saccharine, various fruit flavors and food colorings; *Fritters*—flour, baking powder, egg, and milk; *Gelatin*—cattle, sheep, goat, pig, and fish hides and connective tissues. (See page 74.) *Knox gelatin*—said to be made from beef; *Jell-O*—from beef and pork; prepared flavored gelatin desserts contain sugar, gelatin, citric and tartaric acids, natural or synthetic flavors and coloring.

CREAM

Genesee Royal and Jello Dessert Powders—(butterscotch) granulated sugar, cornstarch, brown sugar, butter, flavoring, salt, artificial color—(vanilla) sugar, cornstarch, flavor, salt, color—(chocolate) sugar, cornstarch, powdered skim and whole milk, cocoa, flavor, salt—*Royal Tapioca Pudding—*

sugar, tapioca, salt, vanilla, coloring, and flavoring; *Ice Cream*—egg, milk, flavors, and sugar; *Ice Cream Powders and Freezing Mixtures*—most of these contain dried milk, egg, cocoa, fruit flavor, salt, karaya gum, coloring in varying amounts; *Ices*—fruit, egg, and flavoring (see Sherbet); *Junket, Danish Dessert*—sugar, tapioca, berry juices, flavoring, citric; *Kremel*—cornstarch, dextrose, sucrose; *Marshmallows*—may contain egg white; *Meringue*—egg, lemon, or other flavor, sugar; *Sherbet*—milk, fruit juice or flavor, and sugar.

MISCELLANEOUS FOODS AND PANTRY SUPPLIES
Pantry Supplies

Baked Beans—beans, pork, catsup, bacon pork, vinegar, salt; *Baking Powder*—alkali, usually sodium bicarbonate combined with an acid such as phosphoric acid, aluminum sulfate, cream of tartar or tartaric acid. Cornstarch is the usual filler to prevent moisture absorption. *Royal, Shillings, K. C., and Calumet* contain no egg; *Beef juices*—meat juice, egg white; *Canned Tomato Soup*—tomato, butter, milk, onion, sugar, salt, flour, spices; *Catsup*—tomato, spices, onions, sugar, vinegar; *Cottolene*—cottonseed oil and beef suet; *C. & H. Confectioner's or Powdered Sugar*—contains 3 per cent cornstarch; *Crisco*—cottonseed oil; *Highland Maple Sap Syrup*—100 per cent maple syrup; *Log Cabin Maple Syrup*—cane sugar, maple syrup; *Jam and Jellies*—fruit and sugar, sometimes contain corn syrup; *Mazola Oil*—corn oil; *Maraschino Cherries*—artificial coloring and flavoring, sulphur dioxide, sugar, corn syrup; *Nucoa—Oleomargarine*—animal or vegetable fat churned in milk; *Olive Oil*—some brands are pure, others adulterated with other commercial oils. (See pages 96 and 97.) *Potato Chips*—usually fried in cottonseed oil, also in corn, cocoanut, peanut or other edible oils; *Salad Oil*—usually cottonseed oil, though corn, peanut, sesame or other edible oils occasionally may be present; *Spices*—described and listed on pages 84, 95 and 96. *Syrups*—combinations of corn and maple syrup and cane sugar; *Vinegar*—dilute acetic acid from fermentation of alcohol; apple or cider vinegar most common; wine or grape vinegar, beer vinegar in England, sugar vinegar from molasses, glucose vinegar from corn syrup, and white vinegar from dilute alcohol; dilute acetic acid may be used by allergics (3 teaspoonfuls of 28 per cent acetic acid to 5 ounces of water); *Wesson Oil*—cottonseed oil; *Worcestershire Sauces*—vary in content; usually contain soy, vinegar, lime juice, onions, tamarinds, garlic, fish such as anchovies or pickled herring, red chili, and spices; *Yeast*—microscopic fungi prepared with small amounts of wheat, corn, rye, or barley malt. Actual ingredients of the brand used may be learned from the manufacturer.

Sauces

Best Foods French Dressing—oil, vinegar, salt, tomato, spices, tragacanth, and egg yolk; *Cream Sauce*—butter, flour, milk, eggs, flavors; *French Dressing*—olive or salad oil, vinegar, salt, pepper, spices, tragacanth; *Girard's French Dressing*—oil, vinegar, salt, spices, garlic; *Hollandaise*—eggs, butter, lemon juice; *Mayonnaise*—olive or salad oil, eggs, vinegar, spices, sugar, and salt; *Miracle Whip Salad Dressing*—cottonseed and corn oil, vinegar, spices, sugar, salt, eggs, arrowroot, and cornstarch; *Tartar Sauce*—mayonnaise, capers, olives, cucumber, pickles, spices; *White Sauce*—butter, flour, milk, seasoning.

Seasoned and Spiced Foods
(For pure spices, see pages 84, 95 and 96)

Chutney—East Indian pickle, usually with mangoes, raisins, tamarinds, limes, ginger, chilis, and other spices. Domestic chutneys contain some sweet acid fruit such as lemon or tamarinds seasoned as above; *Chow Chow*—a mixture of pickled vegetables and mustard; *Curry*—a highly seasoned East Indian condiment, usually containing tumeric, coriander, black pepper, cayenne pepper, fenugreek seed, cumin, ginger and lime; *Enchilades*—corn, wheat flour, beef, pork, onions, garlic, chili, tomato paste, cheese, eggs, olives. *Minced Meats*—apple, raisins, spices, brandy, sherry, rum, sugar, citrus, fruit in varying amounts. Beef no longer included in commercial products. *Mulligatawny*—originally an East Indian soup whose name means pepper water. It usually contains curry powder, meats, vegetables, mango, cocoanut, rice, cayenne pepper, and other spices; *Mushroom Sauce*—tomato purée, flour, beef, oil, mushrooms, onions, garlic, salt, spices; *Tamale*—cornmeal, rice, and practically always wheat and some other flour; meats of various kinds, chilis, garlic, pepper, and other flavors. *Tomato Sauce*—tomato purée, salt, green peppers, onions, garlic, spices.

Meat Products

Bologna—beef, veal, pork, spices, onion. Casings of this and similar products may contain egg. *Calves' Feet*—gelatin, citric acid, sugar, and wine; *Corned Beef*—beef treated with salt and saltpeter, sugar, and various spices such as allspice, coriander, mace, nutmeg, thyme, and sage; *Deviled Meats*—beef, pork, pepper, onion or garlic, cloves, paprika, mustard, coriander, mace, anise, and other spices in varying amounts; *Frankfurters*—beef, pork, at times veal, milk, or cereals, onions, and spices stuffed in sheep casings; *Goose Liver*—calf's liver, pork, goose liver; *Pate de Foie Gras*—goose liver, truffles, spices; it usually contains pork; *Salami*—pork, beef, grape juice, garlic, spices; *Salmagundi*—chopped meat, fish, anchovies, onions, pickles, vinegar, pepper, and other ingredients; *Sausages*—chopped meat, usually beef or pork, cured, spiced and stuffed in beef, sheep, or hog casings; often contain potato, rice, wheat, at times milk and egg; *Scrapple*—pork, cornmeal or buckwheat with spices and herbs; *Tripe*—inner lining of stomach, usually from beef but also from veal, sheep or hog; *Veal or Meat Loaf*—may contain veal, pork, beef, egg, flour, bread crumbs, onion, pepper, and spices in varying amounts. *Vienna Sausage*—pork, beef, spices, stuffed in sheep or hog intestinal casings.

Canned Soups

As stated on page 149, these cannot be used in Elimination Diets unless every ingredient is ascertained from the manufacturer and all have been allowed by the physician. Likewise hotel, restaurant soups, and those in friends' homes contain many ingredients of unknown or uncertain content. It must be remembered especially that consomme usually contains egg and tomato. Cream soups contain cream, butter, wheat flour, and usually pepper.

Spices, Flavoring Herbs and Their Uses*

Column headers (spices):

Allspice — whole, ground
Anise
Basil
Bay Leaf
Caraway Seed
Cardamom Seed — whole, decorticated
Cassia — ground, sticks, buds
Cayenne
Celery — seeds, juice
Chili — pods, powder
Cinnamon — sticks, ground
Cloves — whole, ground
Coriander — whole, ground
Cumin
Curry Powder
Dill
Fennel
Fenugreek
Garlic — powder, juice
Ginger — cracked, ground
Juniper Berries
Mace — blades, ground
Marjoram
Mustard — seed, flour
Nutmeg — whole, ground
Onion — dehydrated, juice
Oreganum
Paprika
Parsley — seed, juice
Pepper — whole, ground
Poppy Seed
Rosemary
Saffron
Sage
Savory
Sesame Seed
Tarragon
Thyme
Tonka Bean
Turmeric
Vanilla Bean

FOODS

Bread and Rolls
Cakes and Cookies
Candy
Canned Foods
Carbonated Beverages
Catsup and Chili Sauce
Cheese
Chili Con Carne
Condiment Sauces
Crackers and Biscuits
Fish (Packed)
Fruit Preserves
Mayonnaise
Meats
Pickles
Pie Fillings
Poultry Seasoning
Salad Dressings
Sausages and Chopped Meats
Soups
Spice Extractives
Spice Oils

FEEDS AND MISCELLANEOUS

Cattle Feed
Chicken Feed
Cordials
Gin
Insecticides
Perfumes
Pharmaceuticals
Tobacco Products

* (Courtesy of Food Industries, **10**, 423, 1938.)

RECIPES

All measurements are level.

Use standard 8 oz. measuring cups and standard measuring spoons.

Since many soy and lima flours are not refined, breads made of these flours have a tendency to become moldy more quickly than wheat breads. This can be prevented if the bread is wrapped in waxed paper and stored in the refrigerator or cooler.

Table of Abbreviations and Measurements

Tbsp.	=	tablespoonful	16 Tbsp.	=	1 cup
tsp.	=	teaspoonful	8 Tbsp.	=	$\frac{1}{2}$ cup
cup	=	cupful	8 oz.	=	1 cup
			3 tsp.	=	1 Tbsp.

The following recipes have been devised for special use with the elimination diets in this volume. When soy and lima flours are required, the product varies according to the type of flour used. The refined flours (see page 82) or the raw or locally ground flours may be used according to the experience of the baker or cook. The numbers refer to the special meals where recipes are used in the diets.

(1)   *Fruit Tapioca*

$2\frac{1}{2}$ cups canned fruit juice and water

4 Tbsp. Minute tapioca

$\frac{1}{2}$ cup sugar

$\frac{1}{4}$ tsp. salt

1 to $1\frac{1}{2}$ cups chopped or puréed apricots, pears, prunes or pineapple

1 Tbsp. lemon juice

Combine fruit juice and water, Minute tapioca, sugar and salt in a sauce pan and mix well. Bring mixture to a boil, stirring constantly. Remove from fire. Cool, stirring occasionally. Mixture thickens as it cools.

(2)   *Brown Sugar Tapioca*

3 cups water

$\frac{1}{3}$ cup Minute tapioca

$\frac{1}{3}$ cup sugar, or

$\frac{1}{2}$ cup brown sugar

$\frac{1}{4}$ tsp. salt

1 Tbsp. lemon juice and 2 tsp. grated rind, or

$\frac{1}{2}$ tsp. maple flavoring and 1 tsp. vanilla extract, or

2 tsp. caramel flavoring

(The amount of brown sugar and flavoring may be varied to suit the individual taste.)

Combine all ingredients in a saucepan. Bring mixture quickly to a full boil over direct heat, stirring constantly. Remove from the fire. Do not overcook. Stir occasionally as it cools. Lemon juice and rind may be omitted if not included in the diet.

(3)   *Lamb Patties*

Ground lamb pressed into small patties. Broiled or fried.

(4–a)   *Soy Bean-Tapioca Bread*

2 cups sifted soy flour   4½ tsp. baking powder
½ cup potato flour   1 cup cooked tapioca (2 tsp.
1 tsp. salt   tapioca cooked in 1 cup water.
4½ tsp. sugar   Cool and add water to make 1
4 Tbsp. sesame oil   cup.)

Sift together all dry ingredients. Add cooked tapioca and sesame oil.
Mix well. Pour into a loaf pan which has been greased with sesame oil
and lined with waxed paper. Place in a cold oven and gradually raise the
thermostat to 350° F. Bake for 1½ hours.

(4–b)   *Soy-Lima-Potato Bread*

1 cup potato flour   2 Tbsp. sugar
¾ cup soy bean flour   1 cup water
¼ cup lima bean flour   6 tsp. baking powder
3 Tbsp. sesame oil   ½ tsp. salt

Sift the flour, baking powder and salt together three times. Mix sugar
and oil and add the flour and water alternately. Pour into a well greased
loaf pan and bake at 350° F. for 1 or 1½ hours.

(5–a)   *Soy-Lima-Potato Muffins*

1 cup potato flour   2 Tbsp. sugar
¾ cup soy bean flour   1 cup water
¼ cup lima bean flour   6 tsp. baking powder
½ cup sesame oil   ½ tsp. salt.

Sift flour, baking powder and salt together three times. Blend the oil
and sugar well. Add the sifted flour and water alternately to the oil and
sugar. Beat well and pour into muffin pans which have been well greased
with sesame oil. Bake at 350° F. for 25 to 30 minutes. Makes 12 muffins.

(5–b)   *Soy-Lima-Potato Muffins With Tapioca*

1 cup lima bean flour   ¾ cup cooked tapioca (1 tsp. tapi-
⅓ cup soy bean flour   oca cooked in 1 cup water—cool
⅓ cup potato flour   and add water to make 1 cup)
4 Tbsp. sesame oil   2 Tbsp. sugar
4 tsp. baking powder   ½ tsp. salt.

Sift the dry ingredients. Blend the oil and sugar well. Add the sifted
flour and cooked tapioca alternately with the oil and sugar. Beat well and
pour into muffin pans which have been well greased with sesame oil. Bake
at 350° F. 25 to 30 minutes. Makes about 12 muffins.

(6–a)   *Pancakes*

½ cup potato flour   1½ tsp. brown sugar
⅓ cup soy bean flour   ½ tsp. salt
⅙ cup lima bean flour   ¾ to 1 cup water
3 tsp. baking powder   1 Tbsp. caramel flavoring

Mix thoroughly, bake on a griddle greased with sesame oil and serve
with Sesame Spread and maple syrup, or syrup made with brown and white
sugar fla vored with maple or caramel.

To make caramel, cook sugar until it turns golden brown. When cool, add just enough water to dissolve the hard caramel. The resulting liquid may be kept in a jar and used as desired for flavoring and coloring.

(6–b)   *Waffles*

½ cup soy bean flour   Salt—1 pinch
¼ cup lima bean flour   ¾ to 1 cup water
¼ cup Swan's potato starch flour   1 Tbsp. sugar
3 tsp. baking powder   1 Tbsp. melted shortening or oil

Sift dry ingredients twice. Add water and beat to a smooth batter. Add melted shortening or oil. Bake in waffle iron, being sure that the iron is fairly hot, or the batter will stick. This amount makes two waffles.

(7–a)   *Pineapple-Apricot Marmalade*

4 cups apricot pulp—fruit cut in   1 cup crushed pineapple—juice
   small pieces and packed solidly   and pulp
   in the cup   3½ cups sugar

Mix fruit and sugar and boil rapidly until thick—approximately 30 minutes. Seal in hot, sterile glasses.

(7–b)   *Cotlemade*

1 quart apricots   Sugar
1 quart lemons   Water

Slice lemons, rind and all, very thin, discarding the seeds. Barely cover with water and cook gently 1 hour. Add the apricots, halved and pitted, and cook another hour, stirring occasionally. Measure the fruit and add an equal quantity of sugar. Boil rapidly, stirring frequently, until the jelly stage is reached. Seal in sterile glasses. This marmalade is rather tart.

(8–a)   *Grapefruit Marmalade*

3 large grapefruit   Water
Sugar

Cut the fruit very fine. Measure and cover with 2½ times as much water. Let it stand overnight and the next morning boil briskly for 20 minutes. Remove from the fire and measure, adding 1 cup of sugar to each cup of fruit. Stir well until sugar is dissolved and let stand several hours. Boil briskly until it jells. Pour into hot, sterile glasses and seal.

(8–b)   *Lemon Marmalade*

Six lemons, unpeeled. Slice very thin and cut crosswise into small pieces. Measure fruit. Add three times as much water. Boil about 1 hour or until tender. Replace liquid boiled away with water. Allow ¾ cup sugar to each cup of fruit juice. Cook in 2-cup lots to the jelly test (thick, reluctant drops from the spoon—about 10 minutes). Pour into sterilized jelly glasses. Cover with paraffin. This makes eight 6 ounce glasses.

(8–c) *Carrot Marmalade*

5 large carrots   Sugar
4 lemons   Water

Squeeze the lemons, removing the seeds and set the juice aside. Grind lemons and carrots together. Add 8 cups of water to the pulp and boil for 30 or 45 minutes. Measure this mixture and to it add an equal quantity of sugar and the lemon juice. Boil briskly for an hour or until it jells. Pour into sterile hot glasses and seal with paraffin.

(9) *Tomato Preserves*

Select firm, ripe tomatoes. Remove the skins, cut in slices and drain an hour or more. For each cup of tomatoes add a cup of sugar and boil until thick, stirring often. Sliced lemon may be added to the tomatoes while cooking.

(10–a) *Pear Marmalade*

Peel fresh pears; slice and cover with sugar, using ¾ pound of sugar to 1 pound of fruit. Let stand until a syrup forms—boil slowly until thick. When fruit is partly cooked, add one-half can of grated pineapple for each 4 pounds of pears used in the recipe. Then seal in sterilized jars.

(10–b) *Pear Butter*

Peel and core 1 gallon of fresh pears; put in kettle and add 2 cups water; boil slowly; when done put through a colander. To every 4 cups of pulp add 2 cups of sugar. Place on stove again and cook slowly until dark and very thick. Stir occasionally. A few minutes before removing, add juice of 1 lemon. Sterilize jars, rubbers and lids; fill and seal while hot.

(11) *Lima Bean or Split Pea Soup*

1 cup split peas or lima beans   1 qt. water
2 Tbsp. bacon fat   Salt
Diced bacon, crisp

Cook the split peas or lima beans and salt until they form a smooth purée. Just before serving, add the bacon fat and crisp fried bacon.

(12) *Salad Suggestions*

(*a*) Tomatoes stuffed with tiny green lima beans which have been marinated in French dressing.
(*b*) Sliced marinated beets mixed with cold sliced tongue and shredded lettuce and French dressing.
(*c*) Cold artichoke served with oil, salt and lemon juice.
(*d*) Cut lemon or lime gelatin into ¾ inch cubes and serve with fruit salads or fruit cocktails.

(13) *Broiled Grapefruit*

Cut grapefruit in halves, remove the center, and cut around each section. Sprinkle a teaspoonful of brown sugar over each half. Place under the broiler and broil for 10 to 12 minutes. Serve hot.

Sliced pineapple, apricots, peaches or prunes prepared in a similar way are attractive and delicious additions to broiled lamb chops, steak or chicken.

(14)   *Fruit Tapioca*

2½ cups fruit juice and water   ¼ tsp. salt
¼ cup Minute tapioca   1 to 1½ cups diced canned fruit—
2 Tbsp. lemon juice   use only fruit included in the
½ cup sugar   diet

Combine fruit juice, water, tapioca, sugar and salt in a saucepan and
mix well.   Bring the mixture quickly to a full boil over direct heat, stirring
constantly.   Remove from the fire.   (Mixture will be thin.   Do not overcook.)   Add the canned fruit and lemon juice.   Cool, stirring occasionally.
Mixture thickens as it cools.   Less sugar may be added if tapioca is used
as a cereal substitute for breakfast.

(15)   *Baked Pears*

6 medium sized pears   1 cup sugar, white or brown
½ cup water

Wash the pears and remove the blossom ends.   Place in a baking dish,
add sugar and water, cover and bake at 350° F. for 1 hour, or until pears
are tender.   Peaches may be baked in the same way, in which case select
firm fruit and peel before baking.

(16–a)   *Lemon Ice*
                      (Made in the Refrigerator)

⅔ cup sugar   Pinch of salt
2 cups water   ⅓ cup lemon juice
1½ tsp. plain unflavored gelatin   1 tsp. grated lemon rind
   soaked in 3 Tbsp. water

Cook sugar and water together together 3 minutes.   Dissolve soaked
gelatin in the hot syrup.   Add salt and lemon juice.   Turn into the refrigerator try and freeze until solid 1 inch from edge of tray.   Scrape from the
sides of the tray and transfer to a chilled bowl.   Beat with a chilled rotary
heater until fluffy and smooth.   Return to tray and freeze again until firm.

(16–b)   *Apricot Ice*

⅔ cup sugar   1½ cups apricot nectar or puréed
½ cup water   apricots and juice
Pinch of salt   2 Tbsp. lemon juice
1½ tsp. gelatin soaked in 3 Tbsp.   1 tsp. grated lemon rind, if de-
   water   sired

Follow directions above for Lemon Ice.

(16–c)   *Pineapple Ice*

Substitute 1½ cups of canned, crushed, undrained pineapple in the recipe
for Apricot Ice.

(16–d)   *Lemon Ice*
                      (Using a mechanical freezer)

1 cup sugar   ½ tsp. grated lemon rind
3 cups water   ½ cup lemon juice

Boil sugar and water for 5 minutes.   Remove from stove and cool.
Add lemon juice and rind.   Pour into the freezer can and freeze, using
6 or 8 parts of ice to 1 part of rock salt.   This makes a little over 1 quart.

16

(16–e)   *Pineapple or Apricot Ice*

1 cup sugar	2 cups canned, crushed pineapple
3 cups water	or apricot purée
1 Tbsp. lemon juice	¼ tsp. salt

Follow directions above for Lemon Ice using a mechanical freezer.

NOTE.—Maple flavoring or caramel may be substituted if fruit is not allowed in the diet.

(16–f)   *Frappés*

Frappés are water ices frozen to mush consistency and may have large crystals through them. Tomato juice, various combinations of fruit juice, or puréed fruits and juice can be used. They may be served as a dessert or beverage.

(17–a)   *Drop Cookies*

¾ cup soy bean flour	4 Tbsp. sesame oil
¼ cup lima bean flour	3 tsp. baking powder
1 cup potato flour	1 cup chopped canned apricots
1 cup sugar	and juice
¼ tsp. salt	¼ cup water

Sift flours, baking powder and salt three times. Blend the sugar and oil and add the sifted dry ingredients alternately with the apricots and juice. The amount of water needed varies with the consistency of the apricots. The batter should be thick enough to hold its shape when dropped from a spoon or a cookie press. Bake at 375° F. for about 15 minutes. If stored in a covered container these cookies remain soft. Crushed pineapple or chopped prunes may be substituted for the apricots.

(17–b)   *Crisp Sugar Cookies*

1 cup potato flour	2 tsp. baking powder
¾ cup soy bean flour	½ tsp. salt
¼ cup lima bean flour	1 cup water
½ cup sesame oil	1 tsp. vanilla or lemon extract,
1 cup cane sugar	maple or caramel flavoring

Sift the flours, salt, and baking powder together three times. Cream the oil and sugar and to this mixture add the sifted dry ingredients alternately with the water, beginning and ending with flour. Mix thoroughly. Drop from teaspoon onto a cookie sheet which has been greased with sesame oil. A light dusting with lima bean or potato flour will prevent sticking. Bake in a hot oven at 375° F. for 10 to 15 minutes. Remove from the pan immediately and sprinkle with sugar. When cool, store in tightly covered container. Sesame seeds may be sprinkled over cookies before baking. By substituting brown sugar for white the cookies will be soft instead of crisp.

(17–c)   *Layer Cake*

1 cup potato flour   1 cup water
¾ cup soy bean flour   6 tsp. baking powder
¼ cup lima bean flour   ½ tsp. salt
½ cup sesame oil   2 tsp. vanilla or lemon
   or Sesame Spread*   extract
1 cup sugar

Sift flours, baking powder and salt three times.   Cream the oil and sugar well.   Add the sifted flour and water alternately to the sugar and oil, beginning and ending with flour.   Add seasoning and mix well.   Divide the batter into two layer cake pans which have been oiled with sesame oil. Bake in a moderate oven, about 375° F. for 20 minutes.   This batter may be used for cup cakes also.   To prevent sticking remove cake from pans while hot.

(17–d)   *Upside-Down Cake*

¼ cup Sesame Spread*   1 No. 2 can sliced pineapple,
½ cup brown sugar   pears, apricots or prunes

Melt Sesame Spread in a skillet.   Add brown sugar and stir constantly, cooking slowly 10 minutes.   Cover with drained pineapple, pear halves, apricots or dried prunes.   Set aside to cool while making the cake.   Use the recipe for layer cake.   Pour the batter over the prepared fruit, bake in a moderate oven (350° F.) 45 minutes or until done.

(17–e)   *Caramel Frosting*

⅔ cup water   3 Tbsp. Sesame Spread
2 cups brown sugar   1 tsp. vanilla extract

Combine sugar and water.   Stir slowly while bringing it to a boil.   Boil hard, stirring occasionally until the syrup has reached the "soft ball" stage (234° F.).   Remove from the fire, add Sesame Spread and vanilla and allow to cool undisturbed until lukewarm.   Beat the mixture until it gets thick and loses its luster.   Spread quickly over the cake.

(17–f)   *Pineapple Filling*

2 Tbsp. tapioca or potato flour   2 cups crushed pineapple—juice
½ cup sugar   and fruit
                                   1 Tbsp. lemon juice

Mix tapioca flour and sugar, add pineapple and lemon juice and cook slowly until thick and clear.   Cool slightly before spreading on cake.   This may be used on top of the cake as well as for the filling.

(18–a)   *Candied Fruit Peel*

Remove the peel from lemons or grapefruit in lengthwise slices.   Place in a sauce pan, cover with cold water, add ¼ tsp. salt, heat slowly to boiling and boil gently until the peel is soft.   Drain off the water.   When peel is cool enough to handle, remove all the white fibrous portions, using a spoon to scrape it out.   Cut rind in thin strips with sharp scissors.

* See page 156.

In another sauce pan combine 1 cup sugar with $\frac{1}{3}$ cup water. Heat slowly, stirring until sugar is dissolved and boiling point is reached. After that, do not stir. Cook to 270° F. (Syrup forms into threads and feels brittle under water, but soft and pliable when removed.) Put rind into syrup and cook over a low heat until it is clear. Remove to a platter which has been sprinkled generously with sugar to cool. Coat with sugar.

(18–b)   *Glacé Fruit*

2 cups sugar $\frac{1}{3}$ tsp. cream of tartar
$\frac{3}{4}$ cup water

Heat sugar and water slowly to boiling and add cream of tartar. After boiling point is reached, do not stir and keep the crystals wiped down from the sides of the pan. Boil to 300° F., or until syrup just starts to discolor. Remove pan at once from the heat, plunge it into a pan of cold water to stop the boiling, and then set the kettle in a pan of hot water.

The dipping should be done quickly. Have small pieces of well-drained pineapple, grapefruit sections, pitted prunes, or thin slices of lemon ready, each one fastened on a skewer or toothpick. Dip each piece into the syrup. When well covered, remove and place on a well-greased platter to cool. After cooling the skewer is removed.

(19–a)   *Fondant*

2 cups sugar $\frac{1}{4}$ tsp. salt
$\frac{1}{4}$ tsp. cream of tartar $\frac{1}{2}$ tsp. vanilla
1 cup boiling water

Measure sugar and cream of tartar into a sauce pan and add the boiling water. Stir over a low heat until sugar is dissolved. Do not let the candy boil until the sugar is dissolved and the sugar crystals wiped down from the sides of the pan with a clean cloth. When the boiling point is reached, cover the kettle and boil vigorously for 5 minutes. Remove the cover, wipe off crystals from sides of the pan and continue cooking without stirring until the medium ball stage has been reached (240° to 242° F.). When done, pour the candy at once into a cold wet platter and let it stand until lukewarm. Sprinkle salt over the surface, add vanilla and beat until white and knead in the hands until smooth and creamy. Put fondant into a glass jar and cover. It will keep several weeks in a cool place.

Use of Fondant

Put a portion of the fondant into the top part of a double boiler. Melt over hot but not boiling water until fondant softens. Coloring or flavoring is added at this stage. Lemon extract or lemon juice and grated lemon rind, unsalted Se-So Nuts (soaked soy beans browned in sesame oil), chopped prunes or glacéed pineapple may be useful. Drop fondant from tip of a spoon onto waxed paper.

(19–b)   *Panocha*

3 Tbsp. Sesame Spread*   1 cup water
2 cups brown sugar $\frac{1}{8}$ tsp. soda
1 cup white sugar

* See page 156.

Melt Sesame Spread in a kettle, stir in sugars. Add water and soda and mix well with sugar. Wipe down sugar from sides of pan. Heat slowly to boiling, stirring until sugar is dissolved. Boil to 240° F., the medium ball stage (the ball holds its shape when lifted from cold water). Remove from stove, sprinkle a dash of salt over top and set aside to cool undisturbed until lukewarm. Beat until creamy. Turn into greased pans and cut into squares.

(19–c)   *Marshmallows*

2 cups sugar	½ tsp. salt
¾ cup water	1 tsp. vanilla extract
2 Tbsp. gelatin	

Mix sugar and water and boil until the soft ball stage has been reached (234° to 238° F.). Remove from the fire. Soften the gelatin in ½ cup of cold water. Pour the hot syrup over the softened gelatin and stir until dissolved. Let it partially cool, add vanilla and salt and beat it until the mixture is thick and white and will hold its shape. Pour into straight sided pans. When firm, cut into squares. Roll in sugar, or if corn is allowed, powdered sugar may be used.

(19–d)   *Se-So Nuts*

Soak ½ cup of dried soy beans in 1 cup of water overnight. Drain the soy beans and fry gently in sesame oil until browned. Stir constantly to prevent burning. Remove from the stove, spread soy beans on paper towels to absorb excess oil and sprinkle with salt. This quantity makes about ¾ cup of nuts.

(20)   *Corn Pone*

1 cup cornmeal	Boiling water
½ tsp. salt	1 Tbsp. Mazola oil

Carefully pour enough boiling water onto the cornmeal to make a stiff mixture, stirring constantly. Add the oil and mix well. Mold into oblong "pones" and fry in hot skillet with enough fat to prevent sticking. When brown on one side, turn and brown on the other side. Serve hot.

(21)   *Corn-Rice Muffins*

1⅓ cups cornmeal	2½ tsp. baking powder
⅔ cup rice flour	1 cup water
¼ cup sugar	3 Tbsp. Mazola oil
½ tsp. salt	

Sift all the dry ingredients together, add the water and oil. Pour into well-greased muffin pans. Bake at 400° F. for 30 minutes

(22)   *Corn-Rye Muffins*

Use the above recipe but substitute rye flour for rice flour.

(23)   *Rice Biscuit*

Made by the Battle Creek Sanitarium.

(24) *Rice Bread*

1 cup rice flour	1 Tbsp. sugar
3 tsp. baking powder	$\frac{1}{2}$ tsp. salt
2 Tbsp. bacon fat or oil	$\frac{3}{4}$ cup water

Sift the dry ingredients. Add water and fat. Bake in a loaf pan in a moderate oven.

(25) *Ry-Krisp*

Prepared by the Ralston Purina Co.

(26) *Corn-Rice Pancakes*

$\frac{2}{3}$ cup rice flour	Salt
$\frac{1}{3}$ cup white cornmeal	2 Tbsp. sesame or Mazola oil
2 tsp. baking powder	Water to make right consistency
2 Tbsp. brown sugar	1 tsp. caramel

Mix thoroughly and cook on a well-greased griddle.

(27) *Lamb or Chicken Croquettes*

1$\frac{1}{2}$ cups cooked chicken, chopped fine	3 Tbsp. quick-cooking tapioca or 2 Tbsp. cornstarch or tapioca flour
$\frac{1}{2}$ tsp. salt	
1 cup chicken broth (made at home)	

Cook the tapioca in the chicken broth for 6 minutes or until the tapioca is clear. Add the chicken and salt. Chill and shape into croquettes. Roll in crushed cornflakes, rice flakes, or crumbs of soy bean bread. Fry in deep sesame oil or bake in the oven for 30 to 45 minutes.

(28) *Corn Crisps*

1 cup cornmeal	1 Tbsp. Mazola oil
1 tsp. salt	1 tsp. sugar
2 cups boiling water	

Mix all together. Pour a very thin layer on a well-greased cookie sheet. Bake 15 minutes at 350° F. While warm, cut into strips and sprinkle salt over the top.

(29–a) *Rice Fruit Pudding*

1$\frac{1}{2}$ cups cooked rice	1 cup canned apricots, peaches, pineapple, or prunes and juice
$\frac{1}{4}$ cup sugar	
$\frac{1}{2}$ tsp. salt	

Mix all ingredients together and bake in a moderate oven for 30 minutes. Serve warm with a pudding sauce.

(29–b)   *Clear Pudding Sauce*

½ cup sugar
1 Tbsp. cornstarch, tapioca flour
  or tapioca
⅛ tsp. salt

1 cup boiling water
1 Tbsp. Sesame Spread*
1 tsp. vanilla or lemon extract

Measure sugar, cornstarch (or tapioca flour) and salt into a sauce pan. Mix well. Add boiling water slowly, stirring carefully to make a smooth sauce. Heat to boiling, stirring constantly until thickened, smooth and clear. Add Sesame Spread and vanilla or lemon extract and serve hot.

(29–c)   *Lemon Juice*

Use 3 Tbsp. lemon juice or a small amount of grated lemon rind added to the above recipe. Add juice and rind last.

(29–d)   *Maple or Caramel Sauce*

Use ½ tsp. maple flavoring or 1 tsp. caramel instead of vanilla or lemon.

(30–a)   *Rice Cup Cakes*

⅔ cup hot water
1½ cups rice flour
2 level Tbsp. shortening
¼ cup sugar

¼ tsp. salt
3 level tsp. baking powder
1 tsp. vanilla

Pour hot water over half the flour. Cream sugar and shortening and add to the above mixture, beating well. Add the other ingredients, mixing well. Bake in muffin pans about 20 minutes in a fairly hot oven.

(30–b)   *Rice Cookies*

3 cups rice flour
2 tsp. baking powder
1 cup sugar
½ cup sesame oil

1 lemon rind, grated
1 lemon—juice of
¼ cup water

Sift dry ingredients, cream thoroughly with shortening. Add grated lemon rind and juice with just enough water to hold dry and pat into shape. Sprinkle with sugar and bake in moderate oven for 5 to 7 minutes.

(30–c)   *Lemon Frosting*

1 Tbsp. grated lemon rind
Dash of salt
3 Tbsp. Sesame Spread*

3 cups confectioner's sugar
2 Tbsp. lemon juice
1 Tbsp. water

Cream Sesame Spread, salt, and lemon rind. Add fruit juice and water alternately with sugar, stirring well after each addition. Place bowl over hot water a few minutes. Remove and spread over cake. This will cover a two-layer cake or 24 cup cakes.

* See page 156.

(31)   *Puffed Rice Candy*

1 cup sugar   ¼ tsp. salt
⅓ cup brown sugar   1 tsp. vanilla
1 cup water   Puffed rice

Cook sugar and water until brittle (254° F.). Add vanilla and salt. Pour over the puffed rice, stirring all the time so that the kernels will be evenly coated. Turn it into a greased pan and cut into squares. Keeps well in an air-tight container.

(32)   *Molded Pear Salad*

Dissolve a package of lemon gelatin in 2 cups of warm water. Pour one-half into a pan and let stand. Fill cavity in each pear half with crushed pineapple, set upon chilled layer of gelatin and cover with remaining gelatin. Let set. Serve on lettuce with French dressing.

(33)   *Rice Pudding With Lemon*

1½ cups cooked rice   1 Tbsp. lemon juice
¼ cup sugar   2 tsp. grated lemon rind
½ tsp. salt   Lemon sauce

Mix all ingredients together. Serve with additional lemon sauce.

(34)   *Rye Bread*

1½ cups rye flour   3 Tbsp. oil
3 tsp. baking powder   ⅔ cup water (more if necessary)
½ tsp. salt

Sift dry ingredients, add the oil and blend with pastry mixer. Add water and stir until smooth. Put in tin and allow to stand for 15 minutes. Bake 45 minutes in moderate oven (350° F.).

(35)   *Rye Coffee Cake*

2 cups rye flour   ¼ tsp. salt
1 Tbsp. oil or chicken fat   ½ cup water
1 Tbsp. baking powder   ½ cup apricot marmalade
4 tsp. baking soda   3 Tbsp. sugar

Sift all dry ingredients three or four times. Combine marmalade with water. Mix all well and bake in a medium oven.

(36)   *Fruit Blanc Mange*

1½ cups fruit pulp and juice   4 Tbsp. cornstarch
1½ cups water   3 Tbsp. sugar

Dissolve cornstarch in a little water. Heat the fruit pulp, water and sugar. When almost boiling add the cornstarch mixed in water. Continue cooking for 15 or 20 minutes in a double boiler. Pour into molds and chill. Serve with fruit or pudding sauce.

(37) *Jellied Prunes and Pineapple*

2 Tbsp. gelatin
½ cup cold water
½ cup boiling water
¾ cup sugar

2 Tbsp. lemon juice
½ lb. prunes—cooked
1 cup diced pineapple

Remove stones from cooked prunes and cut in quarters. Mix fruit, lemon juice and sugar. Soak the gelatin in cold water 10 minutes and dissolve in boiling water. Add to the fruit mixture. Pour into molds and chill.

(38) *Vegetable Chowder*

2 cups diced potatoes
1 cup diced carrots
1 cup lima beans, peas, string
beans—mixed
2 cups stewed or canned tomatoes

2 cups of water or beef stock
2 Tbsp. tapioca or potato flour
Salt to taste
¼ lb. bacon diced and fried crisp

Cover the vegetables and tapioca with water or stock and cook until tender. Dice the bacon and fry until crisp. Add the chowder just before serving.

(39) Use Minute tapioca as a binder in a meat loaf or to thicken stew or meat pie.

(40–a) *Tomato Preserves—Fruit-free*

2 cups well-drained tomatoes—
fresh or canned
Boil until mixture thickens.

1 cup sugar
2 Tbsp. white vinegar

(40–b) *Carrot Preserves*

2 cups shredded carrots
1 cup water
Boil all ingredients until carrots are tender and mixture thickens.

1 cup sugar
2 Tbsp. white vinegar

ADDITIONAL RECIPES*
Soups

Tomato Soup (With Soy Bean Flour)

1 cup strained tomatoes, or juice
1 cup water

2 Tbsp. soy bean flour
1 tsp. salt

Mix this soy bean flour thoroughly with some of the water and add to the hot tomato juice and water. Boil for ½ hour. This resembles a cream soup in consistency and flavor.

* Recipes for wheat-free, egg-free and milk-free bakery products are not included because of space. They can be readily improvised by modification of the various recipes in this volume or may be found in the larger texts on the subject.

Beef Broth (*With Soy Bean Flour*)

2 cups beef stock	Salt to taste
4 Tbsp. soy bean flour	Cooked vegetables

Mix the soy bean flour with part of the stock and add to the hot soup. Boil for 30 minutes. Previously cooked diced carrots, lima beans, peas or potatoes may be added as desired.

Scotch Broth

2 lbs. shoulder of lamb	½ cup diced carrots
2 quarts water	Salt
¼ cup pearl tapioca	

Cut the meat into small pieces and boil until tender. Cool and strain. Separate the lean meat from the bones and return it to the broth, together with the tapioca and carrots. Simmer gently until tapioca is clear.

Hamburg-Vegetable Chowder

¾–1 lb. ground beef	2 cups cubed potatoes
3 Tbsp. sesame oil	¼ cup pearl tapioca
2 cups canned tomatoes	2 tsp. salt
2 carrots—diced	1½ qts. water

Brown the meat in the fat; put all the ingredients except potatoes in a kettle and simmer slowly for an hour. Add the potatoes and continue simmering for an hour longer.

Borscht—Russian Beet Soup

1 bunch beets	½ lb. breast of beef—cut in small
1 cup strained tomatoes—fresh or canned	pieces
1 qt. water	1 Tbsp. lemon juice
	¼ cup sugar
	¼ tsp. salt

Pare the beets and cut them into long strips. Add the tomatoes, water, and meat. Simmer for 30 minutes before adding lemon juice, sugar and salt. Boil for ½ hour longer. Serve very hot.

SALADS

Lamb and Vegetable Salad

2 cups diced cooked lamb	1 cup chopped lettuce
½ cup cooked peas	French dressing

Mix all together and let it stand ½ hour before serving.

Bacon Salad

4 slices bacon—diced	1 Tbsp. sugar
¼ cup white vinegar	1 tsp. salt

Fry the bacon until crisp; add the remaining ingredients. Heat and pour over a bed of chopped lettuce. Mix well and serve immediately.

Tomato Jelly Ring

1 Tbsp. gelatin	½ tsp. salt
½ cup tomato juice—cold	1 tsp. sugar
1 cup tomato juice—hot	1 Tbsp. white vinegar or lemon juice

Soften gelatin in ½ cup cold tomato juice. Add the hot tomato juice, salt, sugar and vinegar and stir until dissolved. Pour into a ring mold. When firm unmold on a bed of lettuce and fill the center with mixed vegetables which have been marinated in French dressing. Use only the vegetables allowed in the diet.

Cooked Spinach Salad

Pick over, wash and cook the spinach or chard. Do not overcook. Drain and chop. Season with salt and lemon juice. Oil small ring molds with sesame oil and pack solidly with the spinach or chard. Chill, remove from molds and serve with French dressing.

Raw Spinach Salad

Wash the spinach or chard well. Leave the small leaves whole, cut the larger ones in pieces. Add ¼ cup French dressing for 4 cups raw spinach. Let it stand 20 minutes before serving. Tender raw spinach or chard may be served in a mixed vegetable salad or instead of lettuce as a garnish.

Stuffed Tomato Salad

Peel medium sized tomatoes, scoop out the center, sprinkle with salt and let them stand upside down until well chilled. Fill the centers with any of the following:
1. Short asparagus tips held with rings of cold sliced beets.
2. Diced cooked carrots and small lima beans.
3. Pineapple tidbits and tomato centers.
4. Pineapple tidbits and grated raw carrots.
5. Diced cold chicken, shredded lettuce and pineapple.

Salad Bowl

2 tomatoes	1 cup cooked peas
1 small head lettuce	1 cup cooked slivered tongue
1 cup tender raw spinach	French dressing

Mix all together in a salad bowl. Chill thoroughly before serving.

SALAD DRESSING

Peach Dressing

2 cups canned peach juice	2 Tbsp. sesame oil
½ cup sugar	1 Tbsp. lemon juice
⅔ cup sieved peaches	

Cook all together for 5 minutes. Chill and serve with fruit salads.

French Dressing

½ cup sesame oil
¼ cup lemon juice or white vine-   ½ tsp. salt
   gar or half of each   1 tsp. sugar

Mix well before using on salads. Tomato juice may be added for vegetable salads or pineapple juice for fruit salads.

Sweet Clear Dressing

½ cup white sugar   ⅛ tsp. salt
¼ cup white vinegar   1 cup sesame oil

Bring the sugar, salt and vinegar to boiling. Cool and add oil slowly, beating constantly with a rotary beater.

MEATS

Lamb en Brochette

1½ lbs. lamb shoulder   3 slices pineapple—drained
3 thick slices bacon

Cut lamb in 1 inch cubes, bacon in 1 inch squares and pineapple in wedges. Place 1 piece of each on wooden skewers, repeating until skewers are filled. Broil under moderate heat until browned on all sides or roast in the oven for 1 hour.

Chicken Pie

2 cups cooked chicken   2½ Tbsp. tapioca
1¼ cups chicken stock   ¼ tsp. salt

Place all ingredients in a casserole greased with chicken fat and bake in a hot oven (400° F.) for 30 minutes, stirring 3 times during the first 15 minutes.

Porcupine Beef Balls

½ cup uncooked rice   1 tsp. salt
1½ lbs. ground beef   2 cups tomato purée

Wash the rice and drain well. Mix with the ground beef and shape into balls. Pour the tomato purée over the meat balls, cover the dish and bake in a slow oven, 350° F. for 1½ hours until the rice is cooked. Remove the cover during the last 30 minutes of baking.

Casserole of Rice and Liver

2 cups cooked rice   2 cups water or stock
2 Tbsp. Sesame Spread   2 Tbsp. rice flour
1 lb. lamb or calf liver   Salt

Line a well-greased casserole with the cooked rice. Cook the liver until tender and cut in small pieces. Make a sauce from the water used to cook the liver (add sufficient water or stock to make 2 cupfuls), and flour. Heat until thick, add the chopped liver and pour over the cooked rice in the casserole. Bake for ½ hour.

Bacon Grill

1 lb. sliced bacon	3 large cooked potatoes
6 slices pineapple	2 Tbsp. Sesame Spread* or sesame
Asparagus bundles	oil

Arrange sliced bacon, pineapple, asparagus bundles and cooked potato halves on the broiler rack. Dot asparagus and potatoes with Sesame Spread. Broil at moderate temperature until bacon is done and fruits and vegetables heated through and browned. Turn bacon to insure even cooking. To serve, arrange fruits and vegetables in center and bacon as a border.

Lamb Tongues

Scrub tongues well. Cover with hot water and cook slowly for 1½ to 2 hours. Season with salt when half cooked. When tongues are done, remove from liquor and skin. Potatoes are good boiled in the liquor.

Lamb Stew

Dredge the pieces of stew meat in flour and brown slowly in bacon fat. As each piece browns remove to hot stew pan and pour hot water into the drippings in the skillet. Simmer for a few minutes and then pour over meat in pan, using enough water to cover well. Cook slowly for 1 hour then season with salt and simmer 1 hour longer. Cook potatoes and carrots and string beans in separate pan. When done combine with meat from which the liquor has been drained. Thicken liquor by slowly adding mixture of 2 Tbsp. of potato flour and cold water. Pour gravy over meat and vegetables and let simmer 10 to 15 minutes.

Spanish Meat Balls

Form ground lamb that has been seasoned with salt into balls. (One pound of meat will make 6 average sized balls.) Brown in bacon fat in skillet and pour canned tomatoes over the balls and simmer for a few minutes. Season the tomatoes with salt. Place in moderate oven and cook for ¾ hour.

Tomato Sauce

2 cups strained tomato cooked down to 1 cup with the juice of 1 lemon, salt and sugar to taste.

VEGETABLES

Dried Soy Beans

Dried soy beans can be prepared in the same manner as dried beans. Cover 1 lb. of soy beans with 1 qt. of water and let them stand overnight. Add fresh water and boil until tender—about 2 hours. The soy beans can be served boiled or baked with brown sugar, bacon and tomato purée, or prepared as a plain purée salted to taste.

* See page 156.

Baked Rice and Pineapple

1 cup raw rice	¾ cup brown sugar
6 slices of canned pineapple or	3 Tbsp. Sesame Spread*
2 cups of crushed or diced pine-apple	1 tsp. salt

Boil the rice in salted water. When tender put it in a baking dish with the Sesame Spread, sugar, pineapple and juice. Bake at 350° F. for 2 hours. Serve with chicken or roast lamb. Brown rice requires a little more sugar than white rice.

Lima Bean Casserole

1 cup dried lima beans	2 cups tomatoes
1 tsp. salt	3 slices bacon
2 Tbsp. brown sugar	

Soak the lima beans overnight. Cook in fresh water for 30 minutes. Drain. Mix lima beans with the other ingredients in a casserole and bake at 250° F. until tender—about 2 hours.

Baked Stuffed Sweet Potatoes

Bake large sweet potatoes. When cooked cut a slice from the top, scoop out the mealy portion. Mash and moisten with 1 or 2 Tbsp. of grated pineapple for each potato, 1 Tbsp. Sesame Spread,* and salt to taste. Fill the potato cases and reheat.

Glazed Carrots

6 whole cooked carrots	2 Tbsp. sugar
2 Tbsp. Sesame Spread*	½ cup water

Make a syrup of the sugar and water. Cook carrots in the syrup, turning often to prevent burning.

Succotash

Combine equal parts of whole kernel corn, fresh or canned, and green beans, lima beans or cooked soy beans.

Harvard Beets

2 cups cooked beets	¼ cup sugar
2 Tbsp. Sesame Spread*	½ cup white vinegar
⅛ Tbsp. potato or tapioca flour	¼ tsp. salt

Make a sauce of the vinegar, potato flour, sugar and salt and add the beets. Serve hot.

* See page 156.

BREADS

Rice Biscuits

2 cups rice flour—sifted twice
4 tsp. baking powder
⅛ tsp. salt

¼ cup cold Sesame Spread*
1¼ cups water

Sift together the dry ingredients. Cut in the shortening. Add the liquid and stir vigorously for 1 minute. Turn the dough onto a floured board, knead for 10 seconds; roll into a sheet ½ inch thick, cut and bake in a hot oven.

Pancakes or Waffles

1⅓ cups rice flour
½ cup cornstarch
1 Tbsp. sugar
⅓ tsp. salt

3 tsp. baking powder
1¼ cup water
4 Tbsp. sesame oil

Sift dry ingredients, add water and oil, beat well with a rotary beater. Bake on a well-oiled griddle.

Quick Sweet Rolls

2 cups flour, half soy bean and
    half potato
6 tsp. baking powder
4 Tbsp. sesame oil

½ cup sugar
1 tsp. salt
1 cup water

Mix flour, salt and baking powder; work in the shortening and the liquid to make a soft dough. Turn on a floured board, knead lightly for less than 1 minute. Roll into an oblong sheet. Sprinkle with a filling made with ¼ cup water, 2 Tbsp. Sesame Spread (see page 156) ½ cup apricot marmalade. Roll up like a jelly roll. Cut in slices ½ inch thick and bake 15 minutes in a hot oven.

Rye-Potato Bread

7½ cups rye flour
1½ cups potato flour
½ cup sugar
6 Tbsp. bacon fat

3 cups warm water
3 cakes yeast
1 Tbsp. salt

Add yeast to warm water, and when melted mix in the sugar, fat, salt and flour. Let the dough rise until double in volume. Knead well with more rye flour, form into two loaves and let it rise again until double in volume. Bake at 500° F. for 15 minutes, reduce the heat to 350° F. and bake for 1 hour longer. If a soft crust is desired rub the loaves with bacon fat.

DESSERTS

Baked Peach Tapioca Pudding

⅓ cup Minute tapioca
4 Tbsp. sugar
½ tsp. salt
2 cups canned sliced peaches,
    drained

2½ cups water and peach juice
1 Tbsp. lemon juice
2 Tbsp. Sesame Spread*

* See page 156.

Combine ingredients in a greased baking dish. Mix thoroughly. Bake in a moderate oven (375° F.) for 30 minutes, stirring well every 10 minutes. Serve warm or cold. Apricots may be substituted for peaches.

Soy Bean Flour Pastry

1⅓ cup soy bean flour
⅛ tsp. salt

4 Tbsp. Sesame Spread*
4 Tbsp. cold water

Sift flour and salt. Chop the shortening into the flour and add the water. Mix into a ball and roll out for two crusts. Bake in a moderately hot oven (425° F.) until it is brown.

Hermits

1 cup brown sugar
½ cup sesame oil
1 cup grated raw carrots
1 cup grated raw potato
2 tsp. soda
1 tsp. baking powder

¼ tsp. salt
1 cup potato flour
1 cup soaked dried prune, cut in pieces
1 cup drained diced pineapple
2 tsp. vanilla

Mix all ingredients together. Drop a small teaspoonful at a time on a greased cookie sheet. Bake at 375° F. for about 15 minutes.

Prune and Grapefruit Pudding

2¼ cups cooked prunes
1 cup cubed grapefruit
1 cup sugar
1 cup prune juice

½ tsp. salt
4 Tbsp. cornstarch, tapioca flour or potato flour
2 Tbsp. Sesame Spread

Pit and slice the prunes. Combine all ingredients and cook until thick, stirring occasionally. Pour into molds and chill. Serve it with the lemon pudding sauce.

Southern Pudding

1 cup grated raw potato
1 cup grated raw carrots
1 tsp. soda
¼ cup sesame oil
¾ cup brown sugar

½ cup soaked dried prunes, cut in small pieces
½ cup drained, diced pineapple
¼ cup potato flour

Mix all ingredients together. Pour into a well-greased pudding dish. Place in a pan of water and bake 1 hour at 375° F. Serve with lemon pudding sauce.

BEVERAGES

Fruit Punch

Freeze 2 cups of apricot juice and puréed apricots in the trays of the automatic refrigerator. Serve 1 or 2 cubes in a glass of unsweetened pineapple juice.

* See page 156.

CANDIES

White Taffy

1¼ cups sugar
⅓ cup water
¼ tsp. cream of tartar

1 tsp. vanilla
1 Tbsp. vinegar
¼ tsp. soda

Combine sugar, water and cream of tartar and stir over low heat until sugar dissolves. Cook without stirring to the light crack stage (270° F.). Remove from the heat, add vanilla, vinegar and soda and mix thoroughly. Pour on a platter greased with sesame oil. When cool enough to handle, pull until taffy is snow white and porous. Twist in a rope of desired thickness. Cool and break in pieces 1½ inches long.

Golden Turkish Paste

1 cup well-drained, cooked apricots
4 Tbsp. plain gelatin
½ cup apricot juice—cold

½ cup apricot juice—hot
2 cups sugar
1 tsp. grated lemon rind
2 Tbsp. lemon juice

Soften gelatin in cold apricot juice. Mix sugar with the hot juice, bring it to the boil. Add gelatin, lemon juice and rind and boil 20 minutes. Remove from the stove and add the mashed apricots. Mix well. Pour into a pan lined with wax paper. After it has set cut into cubes. Roll in sugar or if corn is allowed in the diet powdered sugar may be used.

REFERENCES

Standard texts only are included. Extensive bibliographies of the important articles in the literature are to be found in most of these volumes.

BALYEAT, R. M.: Allergic Diseases—Their Diagnosis and Treatment, Philadelphia, F. A. Davis Company, 1936.

BRAY, G. C.: Recent Advances in Allergy, Philadelphia, P. Blakiston's Son & Co., 1937.

COCA, A. F., WALZER, M., and THOMMEN, A. A.: Asthma and Hay Fever in Theory and Practice, Springfield, Charles C Thomas, 1931.

FEINBERG, S. M.: Allergy in General Practice, Philadelphia, Lea & Febiger, 1934.

HANSEL, F. K.: Allergy of the Nose and Paranasal Sinuses, St. Louis, C. V. Mosby Company, 1936.

ROWE, A. H.: Clinical Allergy—Manifestations, Diagnosis and Treatment, Philadelphia, Lea & Febiger, 1937.

TUFT, L.: Clinical Allergy, Philadelphia, W. B. Saunders Company, 1937.

RACKEMANN, F. M.: Clinical Allergy, Particularly Hay Fever and Asthma, New York, The Macmillan Company, 1931.

SULZBERGER, M. B.: Dermatologic Allergy, Springfield, Charles C Thomas, 1940.

VAUGHAN, W. T.: Practice of Allergy, St. Louis, C. V. Mosby Company, 1939.

17

INDEX

A